Editor
Wolfgang Hiddemann

Handbook of Acute Leukemia

Editor

Wolfgang Hiddemann, MD, PhD
Department of Medicine III
University of Munich
Munich, Germany

Handbook of Acute Leukemia

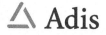

Editor
Wolfgang Hiddemann, MD, PhD
Department of Medicine III
University of Munich
Munich
Germany

Contributors
Michael Fiegl, MD
Wolfgang Hiddemann, MD, PhD
Klaus Metzeler, MD
Karsten Spiekermann, MD
Marion Subklewe, MD

ISBN 978-3-319-26770-8   ISBN 978-3-319-26772-2 (eBook)
DOI 10.1007/978-3-319-26772-2

Printed on acid-free paper

This Adis imprint is published by Springer Nature
The registered company is Springer International Publishing AG Switzerland

Project editor: Laura Hajba

Contents

Editor and author biographies   **vii**

Abbreviations   **xi**

1 Introduction   **1**

Wolfgang Hiddemann

Reference   2

2 Epidemiology, pathogenesis, and etiology of acute leukemia   **3**

Michael Fiegl

Epidemiology and incidence   3

Biology and pathogenesis of acute leukemia   4

Etiology of acute leukemia   7

References   11

3 Clinical manifestations and diagnosis   **15**

Klaus Metzeler

Clinical presentation of acute leukemia   15

Diagnostic testing and criteria   16

Differential diagnosis   20

Additional work-up for patients with acute leukemias   21

References   22

4 Diagnostic criteria, classification, and prognosis of acute leukemias   **25**

Klaus Metzeler

Diagnostic criteria and classification of acute myeloid leukemia   25

Diagnostic criteria and classification of lymphoblastic leukemias   30

Diagnostic criteria and classification of acute leukemias of ambiguous lineage   33

Prognostic factors in acute myeloid leukemia   34

Prognostic factors in acute lymphoblastic leukemia   37

References   38

5 Therapeutic management of acute myeloid leukemia 41
Michael Fiegl

Overview of treatment options   41
Treatment by phase   41
Resistant and relapsed leukemia   47
Treatment of the medically unfit and elderly patient   48
References   49

6 Therapeutic management of acute promyelocytic leukemia 53
Karsten Spiekermann

Overview of treatment options   53
Treatment by risk group and phase   54
References   63

7 Therapeutic management of acute lymphoblastic leukemia 65
Karsten Spiekermann

General approach for management of acute lymphoblastic leukemia   65
Prognostic factors and risk-adapted therapy   65
Clinical trials supporting current treatment algorithms in first-line therapy 66
Overview of treatment options   69
Treatment by phase   72
References   74

8 Future outlook for acute leukemias 77
Marion Subklewe

Emerging therapies in acute leukemias   77
Molecular-targeted therapies   77
Allogeneic hematopoietic stem cell transplantation   79
Antibody-based immunotherapy for acute leukemia   82
Chimeric-antigen receptor T cells   86
Checkpoint inhibitors in acute leukemia   89
Conclusions and future outlook   90
References   90

Editor and author biographies

Wolfgang Hiddemann, MD, PhD, is Professor of Medicine and Director of the Department of Internal Medicine III at the University of Munich, Germany. Dr Hiddemann is best known for his research on the pathogenesis of acute leukemias, and clinical trials in acute leukemias and malignant lymphomas. He is head of the German AML Cooperative Group (AMLCG), the German Low Grade Lymphoma Study Group (GLSG), and founding chairman of the European Mantle-Cell-Lymphoma Network. He is an active member of the editorial boards of several international journals and has been a member of the Steering Committees for the German Society of Hematology and Oncology and the German Cancer Aid. Dr Hiddemann has published nearly 600 scientific articles addressing various aspects of research in malignant lymphomas and acute leukemias. He has been awarded honorary memberships of the Hungarian Society of Hematology and Oncology and of the South African Society for Hematology. He also received the Honorary Medal of the Polish Society for Internal Medicine. In 2003, he was awarded the Charles Burpbacher Lectureship in Zürich, Switzerland, and in the same year the Emil Frei Leukemia Lectureship, Harvard University, Boston. He has also received the Jacqueline Seroussi Foundation Scientific Award.

Michael A Fiegl, MD, is a hematologist and oncologist in the Department of Internal Medicine III at the Klinikum der Universität München, Germany. After attending medical schools in Berlin and Munich, Germany, he completed his clinical training at Munich under the supervision of Prof Dr Wolfgang Hiddemann. He then extended his scientific experience during his postdoctoral fellowship at the UT MD Anderson Cancer Center in Houston, TX, USA under Prof Dr Michael Andreeff. His work has primarily focused on acute myeloid leukemia (AML) both clinically and scientifically ever since; besides basic research on AML and the bone marrow microenvironment, he has collaborated on several large multicenter trials on AML.

Klaus Metzeler, MD, is a senior physician in the Department of Internal Medicine, Hematology and Oncology at the University of Munich, Germany. He completed his clinical training at the University of Munich and studied leukemia genetics as a research fellow at The Ohio State Comprehensive Cancer Center, Columbus, OH, USA. As a clinician-scientist, his research is focused on developing novel diagnostic tools, prognostic and predictive biomarkers, and ultimately more effective treatment approaches for patients with myeloid neoplasia. Dr Metzeler has co-authored over 50 scientific publications on myeloid leukemias.

Karsten Spiekermann, MD, is a hematologist and oncologist in the Department of Internal Medicine III at the Klinikum der Universität München, Germany. After attending medical school in Hannover, Germany, he completed his clinical training in Göttingen and Munich under the supervision of Prof Dr Wolfgang Hiddemann. He received his postdoc education at the Manx-Planck Institute for Biochemistry in Martinsried (Germany) under the supervision of Prof Dr Axel Ullrich. The focus of his work was the pathogenesis, diagnostics, and treatment optimization of acute and chronic leukemias.

Marion Subklewe, MD, is an attending physician and Professor of Medicine with a focus on immunotherapy at the Department of Hematology/ Oncology at the Ludwig-Maximilians-University Munich, Germany. She is head of the diagnostic flow cytometry unit within the Laboratory of Leukemia Diagnostics within the Department of Hematology/Oncology and head of the clinical cooperation group 'Immunotherapy', Helmholtz Zentrum Munich. Prof Subklewe's interests center on translational medicine. Several preclinical immunotherapeutic approaches were successfully translated into early clinical trials focusing on T-cell recruiting vaccines and antibody concepts. She is active in several clinical studies, serving as principal investigator for clinical trials in acute myeloid leukemia (AML) and acute lymphoblastic leukemia (ALL), and as an investigator and steering committee member of the AML Cooperative Group. Prof Subklewe is involved in the Bavarian Immunotherapy Network, the Helmholtz Alliance for Immunotherapy, the interdisciplinary CRC 1243 in Cancer Evolution, the German Consortium for Translational Cancer Research (DKTK), the international Graduate School 'Immunotargeting of Cancer' and the Else-Kröner Forschungskolleg 'Cancer Immunotherapy'.

Abbreviations

ACT	Adoptive cellular therapy
ADC	Antibody drug conjugate
AIDA	ATRA plus idarubicin
AIDS	Acquired immune deficiency syndrome
ALL	Acute lymphocytic leukemia
AML	Acute myeloid leukemia
AML-MRC	AML with myelodysplasia-related changes
ANC	Absolute neutrophil count
APL	Acute promelocytic leukemia
AraC	Anthracycline
ATO	Arsenic trioxide
ATRA	All-trans retinoic acid
BCP-ALL	B-cell precursor ALL
BID	Twice daily
BiTE	Bispecific T-cell engager
BM	Bone marrow
CALGB	Cancer and Leukemia Group B
CARTs	Chimeric antigen receptor T cells
CBF	Core binding factor
CCI	Charlson Comorbidity index
CI	Continuous infusion
CIR	Cumulative incidence of relapse
CML	Chronic myeloid leukemia
CML-BP	CML in blast phase
CMML	Chronic myelomonocytic leukemia
CNS	Central nervous system
CR	Complete response/remission
CSF	Cerebrospinal fluid
CT	Computed tomography
CTLA-4	Cytotoxic T lymphocyte-associated antigen 4
DA	Daunorubicin
DART	Dual affinity retargeting molecule

DFS	Disease-free survival
DLT	Dose limiting toxicity
DIC	Disseminated intravascular coagulation
DIPPS	Dynamic international prognostic scoring system
EBV	Epstein-Barr virus
ECG	Echocardiogram
ECOG	Eastern Cooperative Oncology Group
EFS	Event-free survival
EGIL	European Group for the Immunological Characterization of Leukemias
ELN	European LeukemiaNet
EMA	European Medicines Agency
ET	Essential thrombocytopenia
ETP-ALL	'Early' T-cell ALL
EWALL	European Working Group for Adult ALL
FBM	Fludarabine, BCNU, and melphalane
FISH	Fluorescence in situ hybridization
FLA	Fludarabine and cytarabine
FLAG-Ida	Fludarabine, cytarabine, idarubicin, and granulocyte-colony stimulating factor
FLAMSA-RIC	Fludarabine, Ara-C, and amsacrin
FLT3	Fms-like tyrosine kinase 3
F-SHAI	Fludarabine, sequential high-dose cytarabine, and idarubicin
G-CSF	Granulocyte-colony stimulating factor
GIST	Gastrointestinal stromal tumors
GMALL	German Multicenter Study Group for ALL
HCT-CI	Hematopoietic Cell Transplantation Comorbidity Index
HiDAC	High-dose cytarabine
HIV-1	Human immunodeficiency virus 1
HLA-DR	Human leukocyte antigen-DR
HSCT	Hematpoietic stem cell transplant
HTLV-I	Human T-lymphotropic virus type I
HU	Hydroxyurea
iAMP21	Intrachromosomal amplification of chromosome 21

ICE	Ifosfamide, carboplatin, etopside
IDH	Isocitrate dehydrogenase
IL-2	Interleukin 2
IPSS	International prognostic scoring system
ITD	Internal tandem duplication
IV	Intravenous
LAA	Leukemia-associated antigen
LBL	Lymphoblastic lymphoma/leukemia
LIC	Leukemia-initiating cells
MAC	Mitoxantrone and cytarabine/myeloablative conditioning
MDACC	MD Anderson Cancer Center
MDS	Myelodysplastic syndrome
MFC	Multiparameter flow cytometry
MLL	Mixed lineage leukemia
MPAL	Mixed phenotype acute leukemia
MPN	Myeloproliferative neoplasm
MRC	Medical Research Council
MRD	Minimal residual disease
MRI	Magnetic resonance imaging
mTOR	Mechanistic target of rapamycin
MTX	Methotrexate
MUD	Matched unrelated donor
NCCN	National Comprehensive Cancer Network
NK	Natural killer
NOS	Not otherwise specified
ORR	Overall response rate
OS	Overall survival
PB	Peripheral blood
PCR	Polymerase chain reaction
PD-1	Programmed cell death 1
PI3K	Phosphoinositide 3 kinase
PMF	Primary myelofibrosis
PML-RARα	Promyelocytic leukemia–retinoic acid receptor α
PNH	Paroxysmal nocturnal hemoglobinuria
PO	Orally

PV	Polycythemia vera
RAEB	Refractory anemia with excess blasts
RAR	Retinoic acid receptor
RIC	Reduced intensity conditioning
r/r	Relapsed/refractory
RT-PCR	Reverse transcription polymerase chain reaction.
sAML	Secondary AML
S-HAM	Sequential high-dose cytarabine, mitoxantrone, and pegfilgrastim
SKCC	Sidney Kimmel Comprehensive Cancer Center
tAML	Therapy-related AML
TAD-9	6-thioguanine, cytarabine, and daunorubicin
TCR	T-cell receptor
TKI	Tyrosine kinase inhibitor
TRM	Transplant-related mortality
WBC	White blood cell
WES	Whole-exome sequencing
WGS	Whole-genome sequencing
WHO	World Health Organization

Chapter 1

Introduction

Wolfgang Hiddemann

Acute leukemias are imminently life threatening disorders, which require a quick and precise diagnostic work-up to select the most appropriate therapeutic approach. Acute and chronic leukemias both arise from the malignant transformation of hematopoietic stem cells. According to the lineage from which this process originates myeloid and lymphoid leukemias are discriminated. The discrimination between acute and chronic leukemias is based on their clinical course and their biologic and morphologic characteristics. While acute leukemias are highly proliferative disorders with a rapid progression and symptoms of hematopoietic insufficiency, chronic leukemias have a more indolent clinical course with a late onset of clinical symptoms and morphologically partially maintained differentiation potential (Table 1.1).

The diagnostic work-up for the discrimination between the different types of leukemias is based on morphology, immunophenotyping, cytogenetics, and sometimes molecular analyses (for details see Chapters 3 and 4). For acute myeloid leukemias in particular myelodysplastic syndromes and myeloproliferative disorders need to be considered for differential diagnosis

© Springer International Publishing Switzerland 2016

W. Hiddemann (ed.), *Handbook of Acute Leukemia*,

DOI 10.1007/978-3-319-26772-2_1

	Acute Leukemias	Chronic Leukemias
Proliferation	High	Low
Morphologic differentiation	Lacking	Partially maintained
Clinical course	Rapidly progressive	Indolent

Table 1.1 Basic characteristics of acute and chronic leukemias.

Reference

1   Swerdlow SH, Campo E, Harris NL, et al, eds. *WHO Classification of Tumours of Haematopoietic and Lymphoid Tissues*. 4th edn. Lyon, France: IARC; 2008.

Chapter 2

Epidemiology, pathogenesis, and etiology of acute leukemia

Michael Fiegl

Epidemiology and incidence

Acute myeloid (AML) and acute lymphocytic leukemia (ALL) are rare diseases, accounting for approximately 1.3% and 0.4% of all new cancer cases in the US. While the overall incidence of leukemia has been stable since 1975 (13 new cases/ 100,000 in 1975 and 14 new cases/ 100,000 in 2012) [1], the rates for new AML and ALL cases have been rising on average by 2.2% and 0.6%, respectively over the last decade [2,3].

International and US statistics

The annual number of new cases/100,000 was 1.7 for ALL and 4.0 for AML in the US [2,3], and similar rates are observed in other industrialized countries such as Germany with 5.2 new AML cases and 1.6 ALL cases in 2010 [4], and UK with 4.5 AML cases and 1.0 ALL cases [5,6]. In other words, in these three countries AML and ALL account for approximately 35,000 new cancer cases per year. With an estimated 5-year survival rate of 25.9% for AML and 67.5% for ALL [2,3], these diseases were responsible for approximately 12,000 deaths in 2015 in the US alone.

© Springer International Publishing Switzerland 2016
W. Hiddemann (ed.), *Handbook of Acute Leukemia*,
DOI 10.1007/978-3-319-26772-2_2

Age, sex, and ethnicity-related differences

Both forms of acute leukemia are strongly related to age, but in an inverse manner. While ALL has its peak in childhood, AML is more common in the elderly (Figure 2.1). Accordingly, the median age at diagnosis for AML is 67 years and 14 years for ALL [2,3].

There is a predilection for men with AML (4.8 versus 3.3 new cases) while in ALL, there is no gender difference (1.9 new cases in men and 1.5 in women) [2,3]. Caucasians have the highest incidence of AML while persons descending from native North Americans have the lowest incidence. For ALL, people of Hispanic origin have the highest incidence while the lowest is found in people of color [2,3].

Biology and pathogenesis of acute leukemia

Both myeloid and lymphocytic acute leukemia arise from genetic lesions in hematopoietic progenitor cells. The lineage of the progenitor, in which the lesion occurs, determines the type of leukemia (lymphoid versus myeloid), but there is less security about the exact lineage-specific progenitor cells

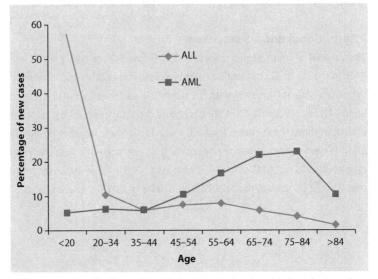

Figure 2.1 Age-related incidence of acute leukemias. Acute lymphocytic leukemia has its peak incidence in childhood, while acute myeloid leukemia is a disease mainly of the older age. ALL, acute lymphoblastic leukemia; AML, acute myeloid leukemia. Adapted from © National Cancer Institute, 2016. All rights reserved. National Cancer Institute, SEER [2,3].

that are affected. Generally, these transformed cells are termed leukemia-initiating cells (LIC) but they do not necessarily comprise hematopoietic stem cells. These LICs represent a small minority within the whole leukemic cell population; both have the ability of self-renewal and modest differentiation (for example, as reviewed in reference [7]). They can be identified by functional characteristics (ie, repopulating potential in mice) and phenotyping of cell surface markers (for example, CD34, CD38, and human leukocyte antigen-DR [HLA-DR]). The leukemic bulk instead, forming the majority of tumor burden, does not have stem cell qualities and hence has no ability to engraft in mice or cause relapse. However, this bulk is responsible for the symptoms of the diseases: overgrowth of the bone marrow with depletion of healthy progenitors and consecutive hematopoietic insufficiency with (pan-)cytopenia and occasional hyper-leukocytosis in the peripheral blood, resulting in organ ischemia due to 'white clots' comprising leukemic blasts and subsequently organ failure.

The genetic lesions that cause the malignant transformation are less well understood. The identification and unraveling of the functional consequences of the translocation (15;17) in acute promyelocytic leukemia (APL) has sparked the hope that for other forms of acute leukemia, especially those with recurrent aberrations such as AML with t(8;21) or ALL with t(9;22), similar genetic lesions could be identified that explain the pathophysiology of the disease and may be targeted by specific therapies. In APL, a balanced translocation between chromosomes 15 and 17 leads to a fusion gene called promyelocytic leukemia–retinoic acid receptor α (*PML–RARα*) gene [8]. The resulting protein comprises a transcription factor that is fused to co-repressors of transcription. As a consequence, affected cells are unable to differentiate into neutrophil granulocytes and remain at the stage of promyelocytes. The systemic administration of high doses of retinoic acid binds the RAR part of the fusion protein, leading to conformational changes with dispensation of the co-repressors, thus re-establishing transcription and differentiation [9].

However, for most cases of AML one single genetic defect is not sufficient for leukemic progression; instead a series of genetic events is required. These events target genes that are involved in different cellular processes, for examples mutations in Fms-like tyrosine kinase 3 (*FLT3*),

K-RAS, or *c-kit* [10], and are supposed to confer a proliferative advantage, while other mutations, for example in *CEBPA* [11], impair hematopoietic differentiation. However, further mutations have been identified that affect genes involved in epigenetic regulation (*IDH*, *DNMT3A*, or *ASXL1* in myelodysplastic syndrome [MDS]-related AML [12]). On average, 13 genes are mutated in AML, only 5 of which are recurrent and these mutated genes can be allocated to one of 9 groups associated with certain biological features (fusion genes, myeloid transcription factors, tumor suppressors, spliceosome, DNA modification, NPM1, chromatin modifiers, cohesins, and signal transduction) [13].

Similarly, in ALL genetic lesions can be found in the vast majority of cases [14]. Best known is the translocation (9;22)(q34;q11.2), which occurs in approximately 15–25% of patients (Ph+ ALL) [14]. This translocation results in the creation of the fusion gene *BCR-ABL1* and confers a bad prognosis. Recently another form of ALL has been identified, which displays a gene expression profile similar to that of Ph+ ALL but without the aforementioned translocation and hence without *BCR-ABL1* [15,16]. This type of ALL is characterized by a bad prognosis similar to Ph+ ALL and was therefore named Ph-like ALL [16]. Genetic characterization has identified deletions in transcription factors relevant for B-cell development (eg, *IKZF1*, *EBF1*, and *VPREB1*) in more than 80% of cases, but kinase-activating alterations were also regularly found, for example involving, among others, *ABL1*, *EPOR*, *CSF1R*, or *PDGFRB* to name a few (as reviewed in reference [17]). In general, these alterations result in, as with *BCR-ABL1*, an activation of intracellular downstream signaling via Janus kinases (JAK; further enhanced by occasional activating mutations in JAK1 or 2), which in turn lead to cytokine-independent proliferation via activation of signal transducer and activator of transcription 5 [STAT5]. In hypodiploid ALL, distinct genetic lesions have been identified that differ with respect to the severity of aneuploidy [18]: while near-haploid ALL (24–31 chromosomes) have aquired mutations in receptor tyrosine kinases, Ras and IKZF3, low-hyplodiploid ALL (32–39 chromosomes) have a high frequency of TP53 mutations. Both subtypes show a high activation of Ras and PI3K, which results in the activation of pro-survival and anti-apoptotic pathways and offers targets for therapeutic intervention.

Etiology of acute leukemia

Even though the exact genetic malfunctions in the hematopoietic stem cells that result in malignant transformation are not exactly understood, several risk factors for the development of acute leukemia have been identified. However, the majority of patients with acute leukemia do not meet any of these conditions.

Exposure to ionizing radiation

Ionizing radiation can result in DNA mutations, deletions or translocations by inducing double strand breaks in hematopoietic stem cells in a dose-dependent manner. The leukemogenic effect of ionizing radiation has long been identified, mainly because of the increased incidence of both AML and ALL in atomic bomb survivors [19] and radiologists that were exposed to high levels of radiation [20]. Similarly, radiation used in the treatment of cancers has been made responsible for the development of acute leukemia [21].

Exposure to benzene

Exposure to benzenes has been known to increase the risk for the development of AML and MDS for several decades [22]. There seems to be a dose dependency, with lower levels of benzene increasing the risk for MDS but not for AML [23], but no definite threshold has been defined that can be considered safe. There is also an association with development of ALL [24], and in many countries, acute leukemia resulting after benzene exposition during work has been recognized as an occupational disease.

Way of living

Besides exposure to chemicals, the way of living can affect the risk for the development of AML and ALL. While the pathophysiological mechanisms are unknown, it has been shown that being overweight [25] and also smoking increases the risk for acute leukemia [26,27]. There is no clear evidence for the role of alcohol intake in adult AML or ALL [28,29], but parental alcohol consumption might increase the risk for the development of childhood leukemia [30,31].

Genetic conditions

There are several genetic disorders that have predominantly systemic manifestations but are also associated with the development of acute leukemia such as Down syndrome [32] and Li Fraumeni syndrome [33]. In addition, inherited bone marrow failure syndromes such as Fanconi anemia and Shwachman-Diamond syndrome pose a predisposition for the development of myeloid neoplasias and acute leukemia [33]. Rare forms of familial acute leukemia also exist, in which certain genes are affected and the families display minor or sometimes no prior hematopoietic abnormalities. In some of these cases, genes are involved that have been associated with de novo AML (for example, *RUNX1*, *CEBPA*, *ETV6*, and *TERT*) but there are also genes that predispose a person to ALL (for example, *SH2B3* and *PAX5*) [34].

Preceding blood and marrow disorders: secondary acute myeloid leukemia

Malignant, but also several non-malignant, myeloid disorders increase the risk for the development of AML, which is then called a secondary AML (sAML). Best known is AML secondary to MDS, and the World Health Organization (WHO) classification recognizes AML with myelodysplasia-related changes as a distinct entity [35]. MDS is a highly diverse group of diseases, and the risk of developing AML varies significantly between the different subgroups. In general, the risk of MDS can be assessed by the morphological subtype (where forms with an increase in blast counts RAEB-1 (5–9%) and RAEB-2 (10–19%) have the lowest survival [36]), but is more accurately reflected by the revised international prognostic scoring system (IPSS-R [37]), which takes into account cytopenias, blast count, and cytogenetics (Table 2.1). With this score, it is possible to estimate the survival probability and to identify groups at a very high risk for transformation into AML (for example, in the group of very high risk patients 25% will develop AML within 0.7 years [37]). Other myeloid neoplasias that pose a risk for transformation into AML include essential thrombocytopenia (ET), polycythemia vera (PV), and primary myelofibrosis (PMF). Chronic myeloid leukemia (CML) in blast crisis, although resembling AML, represents a different entity. The risk for the

Prognostic variable	0	0.5	1	1.5	2	3	4
Cytogenetics	Very good		Good		Inter-mediate	Poor	Very poor
Bone marrow blasts (%)	≤ 2		>2–<5		5-10	>10	
Hemoglobin	≥10		8–<10	<8			
Platelets	≥100	50–<100	<50				
ANC	≥0.8	<0.8					

Table 2.1 The International prognostic scoring system (IPSS-R) for assessment of individual risk in patients with myelodysplastic syndromes. For each applicable feature, the appropriate points are given, which add up the respective risk category (very low ≤1.5, low >1.5–3, intermediate >3–4.5, high >4.5–6, and very high >6). ANC, absolute neutrophil count. Reproduced with permission from © American Society of Hematology, 2012. All rights reserved. Greenberg et al [37].

development of AML in the aforementioned myeloproliferative diseases is approximately 5% [38], but patients at risk cannot be adequately identified, as scoring systems (for example, the dynamic international prognostic scoring system [DIPPS] in PMF) estimate survival in general [39]. Non-malignant diseases can increase the risk for the development of acute leukemia, but the reasons for this are unclear. Among the most common of such diseases are paroxysmal nocturnal hemoglobinuria (PNH [40]) and severe aplastic anemia [41]. However, most patients with these diseases suffer from complications other than the development of acute leukemia but this might change with the advent of more potent treatments (for example, eculizumab for PNH), which will increase survival by the reduction of non-malignant complications (such as thrombosis) but with an unknown effect on the development of sAML.

Prior chemotherapy

While there is no clear evidence that ALL may arise as a consequence of preceding chemotherapy for other cancers, the risk of AML is clearly increased in patients who received chemotherapeutic treatment, for example for breast cancer [42] and Hodgkin lymphoma [43], usually within 3–5 years. As such, cytotoxic agents commonly used in the treatment of malignant diseases have been implicated with therapy-related AML (t-AML), especially alkylating agents (for example, melphalan, busulfan, cyclophosphamide, and carbo- and cisplatin) and topoisomerase II inhibitors (for example, etoposide and doxorubicin) [44]. The majority of t-AML represents with chromosomal abnormalities, which are often unfavorable (for example, complex aberrant 26.9% versus 11.3% in de novo AML [45]) and after topoisomerase II inhibitor treatment mutations involving the MLL gene (*11q23*) are frequently observed [46]. This later form usually develops much quicker (within 1–2 years after initial treatment). The WHO recognizes t-AML as a distinct entity [44].

Granulocyte colony-stimulating factor (G-CSF), given as an adjunct in patients receiving chemotherapy or to stimulate expulsion of stem cells into the peripheral blood for harvesting for either autologous or allogeneic stem cell transplantation, may result in an increased risk of AML and MDS. One large meta-analysis [47] found that in patients treated with chemotherapy, the application of G-CSF increased the risk of development of AML or MDS from 0.4% to 1.9%, however the general mortality in this group declined by 3.4%.

Autoimmune conditions

Patients with autoimmune disorders (for example, rheumatoid arthritis) receiving immunosuppressants have an increased risk for the development of MDS or AML, similarly to t-AML. However, as doses of immunosuppressants including chemotherapy (methotrexate [MTX] and cyclophosphamide) are lower in these patients, the risk of therapy-related myeloid neoplasias is also lower.

Viruses

For AML, there is no evidence for viral infection in the pathogenesis. In certain subsets of acute lymphocytic leukemia, viral infections have been associated with the pathogenesis, for example of adult T-cell leukemia-lymphoma (caused by the human T-lymphotropic virus type I (HTLV-I) [48]) and Burkitt lymphoma/leukemia, which is associated with Epstein-Barr virus (EBV) but also with immunosuppression (for example, acquired immune deficiency syndrome [AIDS]) and co-infection with malaria (see review in reference [49]).

References

1   SEER. SEER Stat Fact Sheets: Leukemia. Surveillance, Epidemiology, and End Results Program. http://seer.cancer.gov/statfacts/html/leuks.html. Accessed August 12, 2016.

2   SEER. SEER Stat Fact Sheets: Acute Myeloid Leukemia (AML). Surveillance, Epidemiology, and End Results Program. http://seer.cancer.gov/statfacts/html/amyl.html. Accessed August 12, 2016.

3   SEER. SEER Stat Fact Sheets: Acute Lymphocytic Leukemia (ALL). Surveillance, Epidemiology, and End Results Program. http://seer.cancer.gov/statfacts/html/amyl.html. Accessed August 12, 2016.

4   ZfKD. Leukaemias (ICD-10 C91-95). Cancer sites. http://www.krebsdaten.de/Krebs/EN/Home/homepage_node.html. Accessed August 12, 2016.

5   Cancer Research UK. Acute myeloid leukaemia (AML) incidence statistics. Cancer Statistics. http://www.cancerresearchuk.org/health-professional/cancer-statistics/statistics-by-cancer-type/leukaemia-aml. Accessed August 12, 2016.

6   Cancer Research UK. Acute lymphoblastic leukaemia (ALL) incidence statistics. Cancer Statistics. http://www.cancerresearchuk.org/health-professional/cancer-statistics/statistics-by-cancer-type/leukaemia-all. Accessed August 12, 2016.

7   Horton SJ, Huntly BJ. Recent advances in acute myeloid leukemia stem cell biology. *Haematologica*. 2012;97:966-974.

8   Arber DA, Brunning RD, LeBeau MM, et al. Acute myeloid leukaemia with recurrent genetic abnormalities. In: *World Health Organization Classification of Tumours of Haematopooietic and Lymphoid Tissues*. Swerdlow SH, Campo E, Harris NL, et al (eds). Lyon: IARC Press; 2008:110-123.

9   Mueller BU, Pabst T, Fos J, et al. ATRA resolves the differentiation block in t(15;17) acute myeloid leukemia by restoring PU.1 expression. *Blood*. 2006;107:3330-3338.

10 Döhner H, Estey EH, Amadori S, et al. Diagnosis and management of acute myeloid leukemia in adults: recommendations from an international expert panel, on behalf of the European LeukemiaNet. *Blood*. 2010;115:453-474.

11 Marcucci G, Maharry K, Radmacher MD, et al. Prognostic significance of, and gene and microRNA expression signatures associated with, CEBPA mutations in cytogenetically normal acute myeloid leukemia with high-risk molecular features: a Cancer and Leukemia Group B Study. *J Clin Oncol*. 2008;26:5078-5087.

12 Devillier R, Gelsi-Boyer V, Brecqueville M, et al. Acute myeloid leukemia with myelodysplasia-related changes are characterized by a specific molecular pattern with high frequency of ASXL1 mutations. *Am J Hematol*. 2012;87:659-662.

13 Miller CA, Wilson RK, Ley TJ. Genomic landscapes and clonality of de novo AML. *N Engl J Med*. 2013;369:1473.

14 Borowitz MJ, Chan JKC. Precursor lymphoid neoplasms. In: *World Health Organization Classification of Tumours of Haematopooietic and Lymphoid Tissues*. Swerdlow SH, Campo E, Harris NL, et al (eds). Lyon: IARC Press; 2008:167-178.

15 Den Boer ML, van Slegtenhorst M, De Menezes RX, et al. A subtype of childhood acute lymphoblastic leukaemia with poor treatment outcome: a genome-wide classification study. *Lancet Oncol*. 2009;10:125-134.

16 Mullighan CG, Su X, Zhang J, et al. Deletion of IKZF1 and prognosis in acute lymphoblastic leukemia. *N Engl J Med*. 2009;360:470-480.

17 Jabbour E, O'Brien S, Konopleva M, Kantarjian H. New insights into the pathophysiology and therapy of adult acute lymphoblastic leukemia. *Cancer*. 2015;121:2517-2528.

18 Holmfeldt L, Wei L, Diaz-Flores E, et al. The genomic landscape of hypodiploid acute lymphoblastic leukemia. *Nat Genet*. 2013;45:242-252.

19 Bizzozero OJ Jr, Johnson KG, Ciocco A. Radiation-related leukemia in Hiroshima and Nagasaki, 1946-1964. I. Distribution, incidence and appearance time. *N Engl J Med*. 1966;274:1095-1101.

20 Yoshinaga S, Mabuci K, Sirgurdson AJ, Doody MM, Ron E. Cancer risks among radiologists and radiologic technologists: review of epidemiologic studies. *Radiology*. 2004;233:313-321.

21 Shuryak I, Sachs RK, Hlatky L, et al. Radiation-induced leukemia at doses relevant to radiation therapy: modeling mechanisms and estimating risks. *J Natl Cancer Inst*. 2006;98:1794-1806.

22 Brandt L, Nilsson PG, Mitelman F. Occupational exposure to petroleum products in men with acute non-lymphocytic leukaemia. *Br Med J*. 1978;1:553.

23 Schnatter AR, Glass DC, Tang G, Irons RD, Rushton L. Myelodysplastic syndrome and benzene exposure among petroleum workers: an international pooled analysis. *J Natl Cancer Inst*. 2012;104:1724-1737.

24 Vlaanderen J, Lan Q, Kromhout H, Rothman N, Vermeulen R. Occupational benzene exposure and the risk of lymphoma subtypes: a meta-analysis of cohort studies incorporating three study quality dimensions. *Environ Health Perspect*. 2011;119:159-167.

25 Calle EE, Rodriguez C, Walker-Thurmond K, Thun MJ. Overweight, obesity, and mortality from cancer in a prospectively studied cohort of U.S. adults. *N Engl J Med*. 2003;348:1625-1638.

26 Pogoda JM, Preston-Martin S, Nichols PW, Ross PK. Smoking and risk of acute myeloid leukemia: results from a Los Angeles County case-control study. *Am J Epidemiol*. 2002;155: 546-553.

27 Fernberg P, Odenbro A, Bellocco R, et al. Tobacco use, body mass index, and the risk of leukemia and multiple myeloma: a nationwide cohort study in Sweden. *Cancer Res*. 2007;67:5983-5986.

28 Pogoda JM, Nichols PW, Preston-Martin S. Alcohol consumption and risk of adult-onset acute myeloid leukemia: results from a Los Angeles County case-control study. *Leuk Res*. 2004;28:927-931.

29 Rota M, Porta L, Pelucchi C, et al. Alcohol drinking and risk of leukemia-a systematic review and meta-analysis of the dose-risk relation. *Cancer Epidemiol*. 2014;38:339-345.

30 Menegaux F, Ripert M, Hémon D, Clavel J. Maternal alcohol and coffee drinking, parental smoking and childhood leukaemia: a French population-based case-control study. *Paediatr Perinat Epidemiol*. 2007;21:293-299.

31 Shu XO, Ross JA, Pendergrass TW, Reaman GH, Lampkin B, Robison LL. Parental alcohol consumption, cigarette smoking, and risk of infant leukemia: a Childrens Cancer Group study. *J Natl Cancer Inst*. 1996;88:24-31.

32 Creutzig U, van den Heuvel-Eibrink MM, Gibson B, et al. Diagnosis and management of acute myeloid leukaemia in children and adolescents: recommendations from an international expert panel. *Blood*. 2012;120:3187-3205.

33 Alter BP. Bone marrow failure syndromes in children. *Pediatr Clin North Am*. 2002;49:973-988.

34 West AH, Godley LA, Churpek JE. Familial myelodysplastic syndrome/acute leukemia syndromes: a review and utility for translational investigations. *Ann N Y Acad Sci*. 2014;1310111-118.

35 Arber DA, Brunning RD, Orazi A, et al. Acute myeloid leukaemia with myelodysplasia-related changes. In: *World Health Organization Classification of Tumours of Haematopooietic and Lymphoid Tissues*. Swerdlow SH, Campo E, Harris NL, et al (eds). Lyon: IARC Press; 2008:124-126.

36 Malcovati L, Porta MG, Pascutto C, et al. Prognostic factors and life expectancy in myelodysplastic syndromes classified according to WHO criteria: a basis for clinical decision making. *J Clin Oncol*. 2005;23:7594-7603.

37 Greenberg PL, Tuechler H, Schanz J, et al. Revised international prognostic scoring system for myelodysplastic syndromes. *Blood*. 2012;120:2454-2465.

38 Frederiksen H, Farkas DK, Christiansen CF, Hasselbalch HC, Sørensen HT. Chronic myeloproliferative neoplasms and subsequent cancer risk: a Danish population-based cohort study. *Blood*. 2011;118:6515-6520.

39 Gangat N, Caramazza D, Vaidya R, et al. DIPSS plus: a refined Dynamic International Prognostic Scoring System for primary myelofibrosis that incorporates prognostic information from karyotype, platelet count, and transfusion status. *J Clin Oncol*. 2011;29:392-397.

40 Harris JW, Koscick R, Lazarus HM, Eshleman JR, Medof ME. Leukemia arising out of paroxysmal nocturnal hemoglobinuria. *Leuk Lymphoma*. 1999;32:401-426.

41 Socie G, Henry-Amar M, Bacigalupo A, et al. Malignant tumors occurring after treatment of aplastic anemia. European Bone Marrow Transplantation-Severe Aplastic Anaemia Working Party. *N Engl J Med*. 1993;329:1152-1157.

42 Pagano L, Pulsoni A, Mele L, et al. Acute myeloid leukemia in patients previously diagnosed with breast cancer: experience of the GIMEMA group. *Ann Oncol*. 2001;12:203-207.

43 Borchmann P, Haverkamp H, Diehl V, et al. Eight cycles of escalated-dose BEACOPP compared with four cycles of escalated-dose BEACOPP followed by four cycles of baseline-dose BEACOPP with or without radiotherapy in patients with advanced-stage hodgkin's lymphoma: final analysis of the HD12 trial of the German Hodgkin Study Group. *J Clin Oncol*. 2011;29:4234-4242.

44 Vardiman JW, Arber DA, Brunning RD, et al. Therapy-related myeloid neoplasms. In: *World Health Organization Classification of Tumours of Haematopooietic and Lymphoid Tissues*. Swerdlow SH, Campo E, Harris NL, et al (eds). Lyon: IARC Press; 2008:127-129.

45 Schoch C, Kern W, Schnittger S, Hiddemann W, Haferlach T. Karyotype is an independent prognostic parameter in therapy-related acute myeloid leukemia (t-AML): an analysis of 93 patients with t-AML in comparison to 1091 patients with de novo AML. *Leukemia*. 2004;18:120-125.

46 Super HJ, McCabe NR, Thirman MJ, et al. Rearrangements of the MLL gene in therapy-related acute myeloid leukemia in patients previously treated with agents targeting DNA-topoisomerase II. *Blood*. 1993;82:3705-3711.

47 Lyman GH, Dale DC, Wolff DA, et al. Acute myeloid leukemia or myelodysplastic syndrome in randomized controlled clinical trials of cancer chemotherapy with granulocyte colony-stimulating factor: a systematic review. *J Clin Oncol*. 2010;28:2914-2924.

48 Tsukasaki K, Tobinai K. Human T-cell lymphotropic virus type I-associated adult T-cell leukemia-lymphoma: new directions in clinical research. *Clin Cancer Res*. 2014;20:5217-5225.

49 Brady G, MacArthur GJ, Farrell PJ. Epstein-Barr virus and Burkitt lymphoma. *J Clin Pathol*. 2007;60:1397-1402.

Chapter 3

Clinical manifestations and diagnosis

Klaus Metzeler

Clinical presentation of acute leukemia

Presenting symptoms in patients with acute leukemia are highly variable (Table 3.1) but most are caused by hematopoietic insufficiency. Typically, the onset of symptoms is acute, within weeks to a few months before diagnosis, except in those patients who develop leukemia secondary to a pre-existing hematologic disease such as myelodysplastic syndromes (MDS) or myeloproliferative neoplasms. Infiltration of extramedullary organs by leukemic blasts is found in 2.5–9% of acute myeloid leukemia (AML) patients. Lymphadenopathy and/or hepatosplenomegaly are present in up to 50% of patients with acute lymphoblastic leukemia (ALL), and patients with T-lineage ALL frequently present with a mediastinal mass. Involvement of the central nervous system (CNS), most commonly manifesting in the cerebrospinal fluid (CSF), is detectable in <5% of adults with AML and in ~5% of adults with ALL at the time of initial diagnosis [1]. Fever is one of the most common presenting symptoms in patients with acute leukemias. Fever should always be interpreted as a sign of infection, and should prompt a careful search for infectious foci. Rapid initiation of empirical, broad-spectrum antibiotic coverage is usually indicated in febrile patients. Fever as a direct manifestation of leukemia without coexisting infection is rare.

© Springer International Publishing Switzerland 2016
W. Hiddemann (ed.), *Handbook of Acute Leukemia*,
DOI 10.1007/978-3-319-26772-2_3

Diagnostic testing and criteria

Recommended diagnostic testing for patients with a suspected diagnosis of acute leukemia is summarized in Table 3.2 [2–4].

Morphology

Microscopic evaluation of peripheral blood (PB) and bone marrow (BM) smears remains the critical first step in the diagnostic work-up of patients with suspected acute leukemia. A differential count of at least 500 BM cells is recommended, and a diagnosis of AML is usually based on the morphologic finding of ≥20% myeloid blasts (see page 25). In contrast,

Signs and symptoms of bone marrow infiltration and hematopoietic insufficiency
• Neutropenia: fever, localized infection (eg, upper respiratory infection, pneumonia), sepsis
• Anemia: fatigue, pallor, dyspnea on exertion, tachycardia
• Thrombocytopenia: petechia, mucosal bleeding, spontaneous bruising, menorrhagia, intracranial or intraocular bleeding
• Bone pain (especially in childhood ALL)
Leukemic infiltration of extramedullary tissues
• CNS: headache, somnolence, confusion, focal neurologic deficits
• Testicular involvement (more common in ALL)
• Hepatosplenomegaly (more common in ALL)
• Lymphadenopathy (more common in ALL)
• Mediastinal mass (T-ALL)
• Gum hypertrophy (more common in AML M4, M5)
• Leukemia cutis
• Soft tissue infiltration
• Arthralgias or arthritis
Symptoms due to hyperleukocytosis and leukostasis
• CNS: lethargy, somnolence, confusion, ischemic stroke
• Pulmonary involvement: pulmonary infiltrates, respiratory insufficiency
• Myocardial ischemia
Constitutional symptoms
• Fever
• Night sweats
• Weight loss
• Fatigue
Coagulation abnormalities
• Disseminated intravascular coagulation
Spontaneous tumor lysis syndrome (rare before initiation of therapy)
• Hyperuricemia, renal failure
• Hyperkalemia, hyperphosphatemia, hypocalcemia

Table 3.1 Presenting signs and symptoms in patients with acute leukemias. ALL, acute lymphoblastic leukemia; AML, acute myeloid leukemia; CNS, central nervous system.

there is no strict threshold for the blast count in ALL, and the diagnosis cannot be made based on morphology alone (see page 30).

If there is any degree of suspicion of APL based on cytomorphology (such as the presence of Faggott cells) or clinical features (for example, prominent coagulopathy or disseminated intravascular coagulation [DIC]), patients should be immediately referred to a center capable of rapid genetic testing using fluorescence in situ hybridization (FISH) or

Diagnostic test	Recommendation
Complete blood count with differential count	Mandatory
Bone marrow aspiration:	Mandatory
• Morphological evaluation of May-Grünwald-Giemsa-, Wright-Giemsa- or Pappenheim-stained slides • Myeloperoxidase and non-specific esterase stains • Iron staining in cases with multilineage dysplasia	
Bone marrow core biopsy:	Recommended/mandatory in patients with a dry tap
• Morphological evaluation (H&E stain) • Immunohistochemistry	
Flow cytometry:	Mandatory
• Can be performed on bone marrow or blood	
Cytogenetics:	Mandatory
• Karyotyping of G-banded metaphase chromosomes	
Genetics (AML):	
• Rapid testing for *PML-RARA* by FISH or PCR	Mandatory if APL suspected
• Testing for *NPM1*, *FLT3*, and *CEBPA* gene mutations	Mandatory in patients with normal cytogenetics
• Testing for KIT gene mutations	Recommended in patients with CBF leukemias
• Other molecular markers	Optional
Genetics (ALL):	
• Testing for *BCR-ABL1* rearrangement by FISH and/or PCR	Mandatory
• Testing for clonal rearrangement of immunoglobulin or TCR genes	Recommended for later MRD monitoring
• Assessment for hypo-/hyperdiploidy by flow cytometry	Optional
Lumbar puncture	ALL: Mandatory
	AML: Optional / mandatory in patients with clinical symptoms suspicious of CNS involvement
Biobanking of pretreatment bone marrow and / or blood	Recommended

Table 3.2 Recommended diagnostic tests for patients with acute leukemias. ALL, acute lymphoblastic leukemia; AML, acute myeloid leukemia; APL, acute promyelocytic leukemia; CBF, core binding factor; CNS, central nervous system; FISH, fluorescence in situ hybridization; MRD, minimal residual disease; PCR, polymerase chain reaction; TCR, T-cell receptor.

polymerase chain reaction (PCR). All-trans retinoic acid (ATRA) treatment should be initiated without delay and before genetic confirmation is obtained. In patients with suspected APL who test negative for PML-RARA, cryptic rearrangements that may be undetectable by standard methods, as well as RARA fusions with other partner genes (ZBTB16-RARA, NUMA1-RARA, NPM1-RARA, and others) need to be considered. In these cases, ATRA therapy should be continued while awaiting the results of cytogenetics and specialized molecular testing.

Immunophenotyping

Multiparameter flow cytometry (MFC) is a mandatory part of the diagnostic work-up for all acute leukemias. MFC analysis and interpretation should follow standardized protocols such as those recommended by the European LeukemiaNet [5]. Specifically, MFC is required to establish a diagnosis of minimally differentiated (M0) AML, megakaryoblastic (M7) AML, ALL, or acute leukemia of ambiguous lineage (see Chapter 4 for diagnostic criteria). Leukemia-associated immunophenotypes (LAIPs) identified at the time of initial diagnosis can be used for minimal residual disease monitoring later on. Flow cytometry can contribute to the diagnosis of APL, which typically shows a CD33-bright, CD34-negative, and HLA-DR-negative phenotype, and high side scatter, however MFC is only an adjunct to morphology and genetic testing in this setting. The blast percentage as determined by MFC should not be used as a substitute for the morphological blast count, or to differentiate AML from MDS [2,3].

Cytogenetics and molecular testing

Cytogenetic evaluation is a mandatory component in the work-up of acute leukemias. Specific cytogenetic alterations can establish a diagnosis of AML or contribute to the sub-classification of AML, ALL, or ambiguous lineage leukemias (see Chapter 4). Metaphase karyotyping allows the detection of chromosomal alterations without prior knowledge of the involved chromosomes or loci. At least 20 metaphases should be evaluated. Metaphase karyotyping is labor intensive, requires high expertise for specimen preparation and interpretation, and is unsuccessful in 5–10% of patients for various reasons [6]. Newer techniques for the detection of larger chromosomal alterations based on microarrays or whole-exome or whole-genome sequencing (WES/WGS) are used in a research setting, but cannot replace standard metaphase cytogenetics in clinical practice yet.

FISH can be used to detect specific numeric or structural chromosomal alterations. FISH is most commonly used to rapidly screen for therapeutically relevant translocations such as PML-RARA in patients with suspected APL and BCR-ABL1 in patients with ALL.

On the molecular scale, advances in genetics led to the discovery of recurrent mutations in >100 different genes in AML [7]. At least one genetic 'driver' event can now be identified in >99% of patients with AML using WES or WGS, including transcription factor fusions (~18% of patients) and mutations affecting NPM1 (27%), tumor suppressor genes (16%), genes involved in DNA methylation (44%), growth factor signaling (59%), chromatin modifiers (30%), myeloid transcription factors (22%), the cohesin complex (13%), and the spliceosome complex (14%). These new insights will change the approach to diagnosis and classification of AML in the future [8]. However, only a relatively limited number of gene mutations have been convincingly shown to be relevant for prognosis, and even fewer mutations have been incorporated into widely accepted and validated classification algorithms [9].

At the moment, testing for NPM1 mutations, Fms-like tyrosine kinase 3 (FLT3) internal tandem duplication (ITD), and biallelic CEBPA mutations should be considered as the minimum requirement for molecular genetic testing particularly in patients with normal cytogenetics, since these markers are recognized in the European LeukemiaNet classification [10]. For patients with FLT3-ITD, the mutant-to-wild type ratio should be reported. In patients with core binding factor (CBF) leukemias, that is, t(8;21)(q22;q22) or inv(16)(p13.1q22)/t(16;16)(p13.1;q22), KIT mutation testing is recommended because of its prognostic relevance. Testing for additional gene mutations should be considered optional in current routine practice, since the therapeutic implications of these markers are unclear. This may change with the availability of novel, targeted treatment approaches, such as inhibitors of the mutated IDH1 or IDH2 proteins found in up to 30% of AML.

Lumbar puncture

Cerebrospinal fluid (CSF) involvement is relatively rare in adult AML, and therefore diagnostic lumbar puncture is generally recommended only in patients presenting with neurologic symptoms such as lethargy, confusion, or focal neurological defects. Imaging of the CNS should be performed before lumbar puncture in these cases to rule out elevated intracranial pressure. In contrast, CNS relapses are common in ALL even in the absence of initial overt CSF involvement, unless CNS-directed therapy is given. Therefore, lumbar puncture is considered mandatory for ALL patients, with intrathecal chemotherapy applied according to treatment protocols. In patients presenting with high peripheral blast counts (for example, white blood cell [WBC] count >20,000/μl) without CNS symptoms, it is prudent to delay lumbar puncture until the blast count has declined. Evaluation of CSF by flow cytometry may increase the sensitivity compared with morphology alone [11].

Differential diagnosis

The diagnosis of acute leukemia is rarely missed in patients presenting with leukocytosis or unexplained cytopenias, if the previously mentioned diagnostic tests are performed. However, in some cases, the differential diagnosis between acute leukemias and related disorders may be challenging. Immunophenotyping is required to distinguish AML with minimal differentiation (AML M0), megakaryoblastic (M7) AML, mixed phenotype acute leukemia (MPAL), and acute lymphoblastic leukemia. Some patients with MDS (refractory anemia with excess blasts [RAEB]) or chronic myelomonocytic leukemia (CMML) present with blast counts close to 20% that place them on the borderline between these conditions and AML. These cases can usually be classified by strict adherence to the World Health Organization (WHO) criteria, although most of these patients quickly progress to full-blown AML. The blast phase (BP) of chronic myeloid leukemia (CML) is morphologically indistinguishable from an acute leukemia. In patients without a known history of CML, prominent splenomegaly may hint towards CML in blast phase (CML-BP). Most CML-BP patients express the p210 BCR-ABL fusion transcript, but there are also rare cases of de novo AML with this translocation [12].

In contrast, the p190 isoform occurs in about 50% of *BCR-ABL*-positive ALL but is rare in CML including lymphoid BP.

Additional work-up for patients with acute leukemias

Recommended pretreatment work-up

Once a diagnosis of acute leukemia has been established, additional work-up is necessary to detect potential complications such as infections and to assess coexisting conditions that may affect a patient's fitness for intensive chemotherapy (Table 3.3).

Medical history, physical exam, including:
- Performance status (ECOG/Karnofsky Performance score)
- Analysis of comorbidities
- ALL patients: testicular exam

Laboratory work-up:
- Chemistry: glucose, sodium, potassium, calcium, phosphate, creatinine, urea, uric acid, lactate dehydrogenase, aspartate amino transferase, alanine amino transferase, alkaline phosphatase, bilirubin, total protein, total cholesterol, total triglycerides, and creatinine phosphokinase
- Coagulation tests: d-dimer, fibrinogen, prothrombin time, and partial thromboplastin time
- Urine analysis: pH, glucose, erythrocytes, leukocytes, protein, and nitrite

Human leukocyte antigen typing of patient and siblings:
- Except for patients with a major permanent contraindication against hematopoietic cell transplant. In high-risk patients, consider early alternative donor search

Active screen for infections, even in afebrile patients:
- Clinical signs and symptoms of infection can be subtle in neutropenic patients

Hepatitis A, B, C; HIV-1 testing

Echocardiogram or cardiac scan:
- Recommended in all patients, mandatory before therapy in patients with preexisting cardiac disease, symptoms suggestive of cardiac dysfunction, or prior anthracycline exposure

12-lead ECG, chest X-ray (recommended)

Consider counseling on fertility protection (eg, sperm or oocyte cryopreservation)

Premenopausal women: serum pregnancy test

Patients with neurological symptoms: CT/MRI of head

Patients with T-cell ALL: chest CT

Table 3.3 Recommended work-up for patients with newly diagnosed acute leukemia.
ALL, acute lymphoblastic leukemia; CT, computed tomography; ECG, echocardiogram; ECOG, Eastern Cooperative Oncology Group; HIV-1, human immunodeficiency virus 1; MRI, magnetic resonance imaging.

Special considerations in older patients

The majority of AML patients are older than 65 years, and elderly patients experience higher rates of complications from intensive chemotherapy, higher treatment-related mortality, and shorter survival. However, chronologic age alone is a poor surrogate for both disease-related and patient-related risk factors. A thorough evaluation of the performance status, by using the Eastern Cooperative Oncology Group (ECOG) scale or the Karnofsky Performance Score, and an assessment of comorbidities using a standardized tool, such as the Charlson Comorbidity index (CCI) or the Hematopoietic Cell Transplantation Comorbidity Index (HCT-CI; www.hctci.org), are strongly recommended [12]. A comprehensive geriatric assessment including physical, cognitive, and psycho-social factors may be helpful for treatment decisions, yet a validated and generally accepted approach is lacking.

References

1   Loeb KR, Cherian S, Becker PS, et al. Comparative analysis of flow cytometry and morphology for the detection of acute myeloid leukaemia cells in cerebrospinal fluid. *Br J Haematol*. 2016;172:134-136.

2   Roug AS, Hansen MC, Nederby L, Hokland P. Diagnosing and following adult patients with acute myeloid leukaemia in the genomic age. *Br J Haematol*. 2014;167:162-176.

3   Haferlach T. How does one work-up an acute myeloid leukemia patient in the molecular era? http://learningcenter.ehaweb.org/eha/2015/20th/103570/torsten.haferlach.how.does.one. work.up.an.aml.patient.in.the.molecular.era.html?f=m6t1576. Accessed August 12, 2016.

4   Döhner H, Estey EH, Amadori S, et al. Diagnosis and management of acute myeloid leukemia in adults: recommendations from an international expert panel, on behalf of the European LeukemiaNet. *Blood*. 2010;115:453-474.

5   Bene MC, Nebe T, Bettelheim P, et al. Immunophenotyping of acute leukemia and lymphoproliferative disorders: a consensus proposal of the European LeukemiaNet Work Package 10. *Leukemia*. 2011;25:567-574.

6   Kayser S, Döhner K, Krauter J, et al. The impact of therapy-related acute myeloid leukemia (AML) on outcome in 2853 adult patients with newly diagnosed AML. *Blood*. 2011;117: 2137-2145.

7   Mauritzson N, Albin M, Rylander L, et al. Pooled analysis of clinical and cytogenetic features in treatment-related and de novo adult acute myeloid leukemia and myelodysplastic syndromes based on a consecutive series of 761 patients analyzed 1976-1993 and on 5098 unselected cases reported in the literature 1974-2001. *Leukemia*. 2002;16:2366-2378.

8   Arber DA, Orazi A, Hasserjian R, et al. The 2016 revision to the World Health Organization (WHO) classification of myeloid neoplasms and acute leukemia. *Blood*. 2016;127:2391-2405.

9   Walter RB, Othus M, Burnett AK, et al. Significance of FAB subclassification of "acute myeloid leukemia, NOS" in the 2008 WHO classification: analysis of 5848 newly diagnosed patients. *Blood*. 2013;121:2424-2431.

10 Vardiman JW, Thiele J, Arber DA, et al. The 2008 revision of the World Health Organization (WHO) classification of myeloid neoplasms and acute leukemia: rationale and important changes. *Blood*. 2009;114:937-951.

11 Bakst RL, Tallman MS, Douer D, Yahalom J. How I treat extramedullary acute myeloid leukemia. *Blood*. 2011;118:3785-3793.

12 Döhner H, Weisdorf DJ, Bloomfield CD. Acute Myeloid Leukemia. *N Engl J Med*. 2015;373: 1136-1152.

13 McGregor S, McNeer J, Gurbuxani S. Beyond the 2008 World Health Organization classification: the role of the hematopathology laboratory in the diagnosis and management of acute lymphoblastic leukemia. *Semin Diagn Pathol*. 2012;29:2-11.

Chapter 4

Diagnostic criteria, classification, and prognosis of acute leukemias

Klaus Metzeler

The currently accepted classification of acute leukemias was published in 2008 as part of the 4th edition of the World Health Organization (WHO) classification of tumors of hematopoietic and lymphoid tissues [1]. A revision has recently been published [2]. The aim of the WHO classification is to define distinct, non-overlapping, and reproducible entities based on clinical features, morphology, immunophenotype, and genetic information. It is important to note that the WHO system is aimed at assigning mutually exclusive diagnostic categories, and not primarily intended for risk stratification or treatment selection. Thus, additional classification systems are useful in clinical practice.

Diagnostic criteria and classification of acute myeloid leukemia

The diagnosis of acute myeloid leukemia (AML) is usually based on the presence of ≥20% myeloid blasts in the blood or bone marrow. In rare cases, the detection of specific chromosomal rearrangements allows a diagnosis of AML in patients with lower blast counts. Table 4.1 summarizes the 2016 revision of the WHO classification of AML [1,2].

© Springer International Publishing Switzerland 2016
W. Hiddemann (ed.), *Handbook of Acute Leukemia*,
DOI 10.1007/978-3-319-26772-2_4

Acute myeloid leukemia with recurrent genetic changes

Detection of one of the balanced translocations included in this category establishes a diagnosis of AML irrespective of the blast count in the marrow or blood. *NPM1* or *CEBPA* gene mutations alone are currently not considered diagnostic for AML. Of note, patients with therapy-related AML who have one of the recurrent genetic changes recognized in this section should be categorized as therapy-related AML. Most

Category	Frequency
Acute myeloid leukemia with recurrent genetic abnormalities:	
AML with t(8;21)(q22;q22); *RUNX1-RUNX1T1*	7% (<60 years)
AML with inv(16)(p13.1q22) or t(16;16)(p13.1;q22); *CBFB-MYH11*	~5% (<60 years)
AML with *PML-RARA*	5–10%
AML with t(9;11)(p22;q23); *MLLT3-KMT2A*	~3%
AML with t(6;9)(p23;q34); *DEK-NUP214*	~1.5%
AML with inv(3)(q21q26.2) or t(3;3)(q21;q26.2); *GATA2, MECOM*	1–2%
AML (megakaryoblastic) with t(1;22)(p13;q13); *RBM15-MKL1*	only in infants
AML with mutated *NPM1*	25–35%
AML with biallelic mutations of *CEBPA*	6–10%
Provisional entity: AML with BCR-ABL1	
Provisional entity: AML with mutated RUNX1	
Acute myeloid leukemia with myelodysplasia-related changes	25–35%
Therapy-related myeloid neoplasms	10–20%
Acute myeloid leukemia, not otherwise specified:	
AML with minimal differentiation (FAB: AML M0)	<5%
AML without maturation (FAB AML M1)	5–10%
AML with maturation (FAB AML M2)	~10%
Acute myelomonocytic leukemia (FAB AML M4)	5–10%
Acute monocytic/monoblastic leukemia (FAB AML M5a/ M5b)	<5%
Pure erythroid leukemia (FAB M6)	<5%
Acute megakaryoblastic leukemia (FAB M7)	<5%
Acute basophilic leukemia	<1%
Acute panmyelosis with myelofibrosis	<1%
Myeloid sarcoma	
Myeloid proliferations related to Down syndrome	
Transient abnormal myelopoiesis	
Myeloid leukemia associated with down syndrome	

Table 4.1 World Health Organization classification of acute myeloid leukemia. Adapted from © American Society of Hematology, 2016. All rights reserved. Arber et al [2].

of the balanced translocations recognized here also have prognostic relevance (see page 34).

Many of the recurrent genetic changes associate with specific morphologic or immunophenotypic characteristics. Patients with *RUNX1-RUNX1T1* rearrangement commonly have AML with maturation (FAB M2), Auer rods, and show co-expression of CD19, and in some cases CD7 and CD56. AML with *CBFB-MYH11* fusion typically shows myelomonocytic morphology with abnormal marrow eosinophils (FAB M4eo) and co-expression of CD2. Patients with *KMT2A* (formerly mixed lineage leukemia [MLL]) rearrangement often have myelomonocytic differentiation (FAB M4/M5) and express the proteoglycan antigen NG2 recognized by the 7.1 monoclonal antibody. The *DEK-NUP214* fusion often associates with basophilia and multi-lineage dysplasia in a hypocellular marrow, and two thirds of patients have *FLT3-ITD*. AML with GATA2;MECOM rearrangement is often characterized by dysplastic megakaryocytes and thrombocytosis.

In the 2016 WHO classification, AML with mutations in NPM1 or biallelic *CEBPA* mutations are recognized as distinct entities, and AML with *BCR-ABL1* or *RUNX1* mutations are introduced as new 'provisional entities' based on their frequency, clinical features, and prognostic significance (see page 34). *FLT3* mutations, although prognostically relevant, do not define a separate category since they frequently occur alongside other changes (for example, *NPM1* mutations, *PML-RARA*, or *DEK-NUP214*).

Acute myeloid leukemia with myelodysplasia-related changes

AML with myelodysplasia-related changes (AML-MRC) comprises 25–35% of adult AML patients. This type of leukemia is diagnosed in patients with ≥20% blasts in the bone marrow or blood who fulfill ≥1 of the following criteria:

- History of previous myelodysplastic syndrome (MDS) or MDS/myeloproliferative neoplasm (MPN)
- Presence of an MDS-associated cytogenetic abnormality (Table 4.2.)
- Multi-lineage dysplasia (dysplasia in ≥50% of the cells in ≥2 lineages)

Patients with balanced translocations listed under 'AML with recurrent genetic abnormalities', *NPM1* mutations, or biallelic *CEBPA* mutations should be classified as such, regardless of multi-lineage dysplasia or MDS history. Patients with a history of cytotoxic therapy or irradiation for an unrelated disease should be classified as 'therapy-related AML' (t-AML). On average, patients with AML-MRC are older than de novo AML patients, achieve lower remission rates, and have a shorter overall survival rate. More specifically, MDS-related cytogenetic changes and/or a history of MDS or MDS/MPN can be associated with an inferior prognosis, whereas the presence of isolated multi-lineage dysplasia (without the other two criteria) seems to have no independent prognostic significance [3]. Recent data suggest that AML-MRC may be genetically distinct from other categories of AML [4].

Therapy-related myeloid neoplasms

A history of previous cytotoxic or radiation therapy is present in 7–10% of AML patients in clinical trials, although this proportion may be higher in the general population. The WHO classification combines t-AML, t-MDS, and t-MDS/MPN into one category since most of these

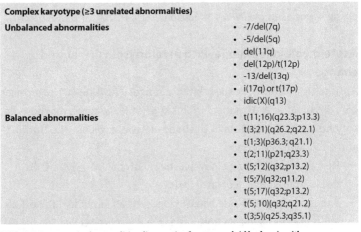

Complex karyotype (≥3 unrelated abnormalities)	
Unbalanced abnormalities	• -7/del(7q)
	• -5/del(5q)
	• del(11q)
	• del(12p)/t(12p)
	• -13/del(13q)
	• i(17q) or t(17p)
	• idic(X)(q13)
Balanced abnormalities	• t(11;16)(q23.3;p13.3)
	• t(3;21)(q26.2;q22.1)
	• t(1;3)(p36.3; q21.1)
	• t(2;11)(p21;q23.3)
	• t(5;12)(q32;p13.2)
	• t(5;7)(q32;q11.2)
	• t(5;17)(q32;p13.2)
	• t(5; 10)(q32;q21.2)
	• t(3;5)(q25.3;q35.1)

Table 4.2 Cytogenetic abnormalities diagnostic of acute myeloid leukemia with myelodysplasia-related changes. Adapted from © American Society of Hematology, 2016. Arber et al [2].

patients have dysplastic features, and t-MDS frequently undergoes rapid progression to t-AML.

All patients with previous cytotoxic therapy or radiotherapy for prior neoplastic or non-neoplastic disorders are included in the therapy-related myeloid neoplasm (t-MN) category, regardless of clinical features, genetics, latency period, or proven causality. Due to the introduction of classes of antineoplastic substances with novel mechanisms of action (for example, tyrosine kinase inhibitors and immunomodulatory substances), the definition of t-MN has become blurred and will need to be revised in the future. Overall, patients with t-MN have an unfavorable prognosis, which is only partly explained by the high incidence of adverse genetic features. Cumulative toxicity of previous threatment and AML chemotherapy may contribute to this observation [5].

Two subsets of t-MN are frequently described: t-MN following treatment with irradiation or alkylating agents are characterized by a relatively long latency (5–10 years), multi-lineage dysplasia, and frequent unbalanced or complex chromosome abnormalities. In contrast, t-MN after exposure to topoisomerase II inhibitors or anthracyclines occur after a shorter latency (1–5 years) and frequently show balanced rearrangements of the *KMT2A* (*MLL*) gene. Core binding factor translocations (*RUNX1-RUNX1T1* and *CBFB-MYH11*) are also observed occasionally, and associate with relatively favorable outcomes [6].

Acute myeloid leukemia, not otherwise specified

AML patients that do not fit into one of the previous categories are categorized as AML, not otherwise specified (NOS), and sub-classified according to their morphology, similar to the prior French-American-British (FAB) classification. These morphological subcategories have no independent prognostic relevance [7].

Rare entities

Myeloid sarcoma (granulocytic sarcoma, chloroma) is a rare extramedullary tumor (<1% of AML) consisting of immature myeloid cells and leading to destruction of the normal tissue architecture, without morphological evidence of AML in the bone marrow. The most commonly affected organs are the skin (also known as leukemia cutis), lymph nodes, mammary gland, testes, and spleen. Myeloid sarcoma is considered to be an extramedullary presentation of a systemic disease, and without treatment, progression to AML will occur almost invariably. A myeloid sarcoma is evidence of relapse in a patient with previously treated AML, and indicates evolution to AML in a patient with pre-existing MDS, MDS/MPN, or MPN [8]. Standard AML chemotherapy is recommended for myeloid sarcoma. Radiotherapy can achieve local disease control but its effect on overall survival is unclear. Radiotherapy can be considered if there is compression of vital organs or residual disease after chemotherapy [9].

Blastic plasmacytoid dentritic cell neoplasm is a rare disease mainly affecting older men (median age ~60 years), characterized by singular or multiple cutaneous noduli with secondary generalization, or more rarely by a primary leukemic course with or without skin involvement. Case series suggest that the prognosis is very poor.

Outlook: the 2016 revision of the World Health Organization classification

An updated version of the WHO classification is due to be released in 2016. With regard to AML, proposed changes include the recognition of AML with *NPM1* mutation and AML with biallelic (but not monoallelic) *CEBPA* mutation as definite, rather than provisional entities. AML with *RUNX1* mutation and AML with *BCR-ABL* gene fusion are considered as new provisional entities. Hereditary syndromes with a propensity to develop AML or other myeloid neoplasms are proposed to form a distinct category [2].

Diagnostic criteria and classification of lymphoblastic leukemias

The diagnosis of the precursor lymphoid neoplasms, acute lymphoblastic leukemia (ALL) and lymphoblastic lymphoma (LBL), is based on a combination of morphology and immunophenotyping. Table 4.3 provides an overview of the most important immunophenotypic markers used in the diagnosis and subtyping of ALL. There is no generally accepted diagnostic threshold for the percentage of bone marrow blasts required to make a diagnosis of ALL. In fact, there is a continuum of clinical presentations ranging from patients with extensive bone marrow and peripheral blood involvement (ALL) to rarer patients who have nodal or extranodal mass lesions with no or minimal bone marrow and peripheral blood involvement (LBL). An arbitrary cut-off of ≥25% bone marrow blasts is often used to separate ALL from LBL. The 2016 WHO classification of B- and T-ALL is summarized in Table 4.4.

B-cell lymphoblastic leukemia/lymphoma with recurrent genetic abnormalities

Within this category, B-cell precursor ALL (BCP-ALL) with *BCR-ABL1* rearrangement needs to be recognized due to its prognostic and therapeutic relevance. *BCR-ABL*-positive ALL becomes more common with increasing age, and often shows a characteristic immunophenotype (CD19+, CD10+, CD25+ with co-expression of myeloid antigens). ALL with *KMT2A* rearrangement most commonly occurs in the first year of life or in adolescents and adults while the *ETV6-RUNX1* fusion and hyperdiploid ALL are frequent in children, but very rare in infants. Patients with *IL3-IGH* rearrangement often have reactive eosinophilia as the gene fusion leads to interleukin 3 (IL-3) overexpression. The bone marrow blast count for patients with this rearrangement may be <20% and blasts may be absent in the periphery.

B-lineage ALL	CD10	CD19	cCD22	cCD79a	TDT	Ig	PAX5
Early precursor (pro-B-ALL)	–	+	+	+	+	–	+
Common (cALL)	+	+	+	+	+	–	+
Pre-B-ALL	+/–	+	+	+	+	c-μ	+
T-lineage ALL	CD1a	CD2	CD3	CD4	CD7	CD8	CD34
Pro-T	–	–	c	–	+	–	+/–
Pre-T	–	+	c	–	+	–	+/–
Cortical T	+	+	c	+	+	+	–
Medullary T	-	+	c, s	+/–	+	+/–	–

Table 4.3 Immunophenotypic markers in the diagnosis of acute lymphoblastic leukemia. ALL, acute lymphoblastic leukemia; c, cytoplasmic; s, surface expression; c-μ, cytoplasmatic μ chains. Reproduced with permission from © Elsevier, 2008. All rights reserved. McGregor et al [10].

Category	Frequency (adults)	Frequency (children)
B-lymphoblastic leukemia/lymphoma with recurrent genetic abnormalities:		
t(9;22)(q34.1;q11.2); BCR-ABL1	25%	2–4%
t(v;11q23.3); KMT2A (MLL)-rearranged	10%	mainly in infants
t(12;21)(p13;q22); ETV6-RUNX1 (TEL-AML1)	2%	25%
hyperdiploidy (>50 chromosomes)	7%	25%
hypodiploidy (<46 chromosomes)	2–5%	1–5%
t(5;14)(q31;q32); IL3-IGH	<1%	<1%
t(1;19)(q23;p13.3); TCF3-PBX1	1–3%	6%
Provisional entity: B lymphoblastic leukemia/lymphoma, BCR-ABL1-like		
Provisional entity: B lymphoblastic leukemia/lymphoma with intrachromosomal amplification of chromosome 21 (iAMP21)		
B-lymphoblastic leukemia/lymphoma, NOS		
T-lymphoblastic leukemia/lymphoma		
Provisional entity: Early T-cell precursor (ETP) lymphoblastic leukemia		

Table 4.4 World Health Organization classification of acute lymphoblastic leukemias. NOS, not otherwise specified. Adapted from © American Society of Hematology, 2016. All rights reserved. Arber et al [2].

Recent developments in acute lymphoblastic leukemia

Since the publication of the 4th edition of the WHO classification in 2008, novel subsets of ALL with potential clinical relevance have been described [10]. These will be included as novel provisional entities in the upcoming 2016 WHO classification.

- Ph-like ALL: A subgroup with BCR-ABL-negative B-cell progenitor ALL have a gene expression profile similar to BCR-ABL-positive patients. This BCR-ABL-like (or Ph-like) phenotype is most commonly seen in adolescents and young adults, and associates with inferior outcomes. Patients frequently have IKZF1 gene alterations, CRLF2 gene rearrangements, and mutations in signaling pathways that might be targetable by tyrosine kinase inhibitors [11].
- iAMP21: Intrachromosomal amplification of chromosome 21 (iAMP21) is observed in approximately 2–5% of children with B-precursor ALL and is also associated with poor outcomes.

- ETP-ALL: A subgroup of patients within the 'early' T-cell ALL/ lymphoblastic leukemia (LBL) category have a phenotype similar to thymic early T-cell precursors (ETP) (CD1a negative, CD8 negative, CD5 negative/dim, and positive for one or more stem cell or myeloid antigens). ETP ALL accounts for 11–12% of childhood and ~7% of adult T-cell ALL/LBL and is associated with poorer outcomes in children and adults.

Diagnostic criteria and classification of acute leukemias of ambiguous lineage

The WHO category of 'acute leukemias of ambiguous lineage' (Table 4.5) comprises acute undifferentiated leukemias (AUL) as well as mixed phenotype acute leukemias (MPAL). Leukemias of ambiguous lineage are rare (<4% of acute leukemias). The diagnosis rests on immunophenotyping. The MPAL group combines the older categories of bilineage (two distinct blast populations) and biphenotypic (co-expression of markers of several lineages on a more or less homogenous cell population) acute leukemias. AUL represents very rare cases of leukemias where no lineage markers are present. Other rare entities such as basophilic or natural killer (NK)-cell precursor neoplasms and blastic plasmacytoid dendritic cell neoplasms as well as non-hematologic tumors need to be carefully ruled out in such patients.

MPAL must be differentiated from AML or ALL with cross-lineage antigen expression. The WHO adopted more stringent criteria to define involvement of more than one lineage compared with the older European

Acute undifferentiated leukemia
Mixed phenotype acute leukemia
MPAL with t(9;22)(q34;q11.2); *BCR-ABL1*
MPAL with t(v;11q23); *KMT2A (MLL)*-rearranged
MPAL, B-myeloid, NOS
MPAL, T-myeloid, NOS
Provisional entity: natural killer (NK) cell lymphoblastic leukemia/lymphoma

Table 4.5 World Health Organization classification of acute leukemias of ambiguous lineage. MLL, mixed lineage leukemia; MPAL, mixed phenotype acute leukemia; NOS, not otherwise specified. Adapted from © American Society of Hematology, 2016. All rights reserved. Arber et al [2].

Group for the Immunological Characterization of Leukemias (EGIL) classification that is still in use [12]. According to the WHO, MPAL is defined by expression of myeloperoxidase (by immunophenotyping or cytochemistry) or at least two monocyte markers (CD11c, CD14, CD64, lysozyme, NSE). T-cell lineage is defined based on surface or strong cytoplasmic CD3 expression, and B-cell lineage is defined by strong CD19 expression with strong expression of at least one other B-cell marker (CD79a, cCD22, CD10), or weak expression of CD19 with strong expression of two of the other markers. Of note, MPAL with *BCR-ABL1* rearrangement is recognized as a distinct entity. Patients with CML in blast phase can also show an MPAL phenotype but should be categorized as CML.

Prognostic factors in acute myeloid leukemia

Prognosis in AML is determined by disease-related and patient-related factors. Older age and the results of cytogenetic testing are commonly regarded as the most important risk factors in AML, and gene mutations have been increasingly recognized as additional risk markers. While the relative frequency of unfavorable genetic features increases with age, this fact alone does not fully explain the inferior outcomes of older patients. Other factors such as comorbidities and poorer tolerability of intensive chemotherapy may play a role here.

Medical Research Council classification

The most comprehensive study on the prognostic relevance of chromosomal alterations has been published by the British Medical Research Council study group [13]. Based on an analysis of overall survival in patients <60 years of age, the MRC classification delineates three prognostic subgroups (Table 4.6). The prognostic relevance of some less frequent alterations is uncertain in older patients.

European LeukemiaNet classification

An expert group on behalf of the European LeukemiaNet has published a classification based on cytogenetics and gene mutations in *NPM1*, *FLT3* (internal tandem dupications, *ITD*), and *CEBPA*, which was subsequently shown to delineate prognostically distinct subgroups in younger (<60 years) and older (≥60 years), intensively treated patients (Table 4.7) [14,15]. Of note, the European LeukemiaNet Intermediate-I and Intermediate-II subgroups do not represent a prognostic grading. In fact, younger patients in the Intermediate-II subgroups have better outcomes than those with Intermediate-I genetics. While the European LeukemiaNet guidelines included all cytogenetically normal patients with mutated *CEBPA* in the 'favorable' group, it has now been shown that only biallelic *CEBPA* mutations are prognostically favorable [16].

Gene mutations

Mutations in *NPM1*, biallelic *CEBPA* mutations, and *FLT3-ITD* are the most well-established molecular risk markers in AML, and are included in the European LeukemiaNet classification (page 34) [15]. Mutations in other genes including *TP53*, *RUNX1*, *DNMT3A*, *IDH1/IDH2*, and *ASXL1* have been shown to be prognostic, but their role in clinical decision-making is not yet well defined [17–19]. *KIT* gene mutations associate with shorter relapse-free survival in the subgroup of patients with core binding factor

MRC prognostic group	Alterations
Favorable*	t(15;17)(q22;q21)
	t(8;21)(q22;q22)
	inv(16)(p13q22) or t(16;16)(p13;q22)
Intermediate	Entities not classified as favorable or adverse, including cytogenetically normal AML
Adverse	abn(3q) [excluding t(3;5)(q21~25;q31~35)]
	inv(3)(q21q26) or t(3;3)(q21;q26)
	−5, add(5q), del(5q)
	−7, add(7q), del(7q)
	t(6;11)(q27;q23),
	t(10;11)(p11~13;q23)
	t(v;11q23) [excluding t(9;11)(p21~22;q23) and t(11;19)(q23;p13)]
	t(9;22)(q34;q11)
	−17/abn(17p)
	Complex (≥4 unrelated abnormalities)

Table 4.6 Medical Research Council classification. *Patients with these alterations are always classified as favorable, irrespective of additional alterations listed in the adverse section. AML, acute myeloid leukemia; MRC, Medical Research Council. Adapted from © American Society of Hematology, 2010. All rights reserved. Grimwade et al [13].

leukemias, particularly t(8;21)(q22;q22), less well established in patients with inv(16)(p13.1q22) or t(16;16)(p13.1;q22).

Other risk factors and prognostic scoring systems

Besides age and genetic markers, a number of other risk markers have been identified including comorbidities/performance status, therapy-related AML, and a prior history of MDS. Various scoring systems have been developed that integrate various risk factors and may contribute to therapeutic decision-making, particularly in older patients [20]. For example, a score based on seven clinical and laboratory parameters, with or without information on cytogenetics and molecular markers, can be used to predict the chance of response to induction therapy and the risk of early death in patients ≥60 years (www.aml-score.org) [21].

ELN genetic group	Alterations
Favorable	t(8;21)(q22;q22); *RUNX1-RUNX1T1*
	inv(16)(p13.1q22) or t(16;16)(p13.1;q22); *CBFB-MYH11*
	Cytogenetically normal AML, mutated *NPM1* without *FLT3-ITD*
	Cytogenetically normal AML, mutated *CEBPA**
Intermediate-I	Cytogenetically normal AML, mutated *NPM1* and *FLT3-ITD*
	Cytogenetically normal AML, wild-type *NPM1* and *FLT3-ITD*
	Cytogenetically normal AML, wild-type *NPM1* without *FLT3-ITD*
Intermediate-II	t(9;11)(p22;q23); *MLLT3-KMT2A*
	Cytogenetic abnormalities not classified as favorable or adverse
Adverse	inv(3)(q21q26.2) or t(3;3)(q21;q26.2); *GATA2, MECOM*
	t(6;9)(p23;q34); *DEK-NUP214*
	t(v;11)(v;q23); *KMT2A (MLL)*-rearranged [except t(9;11)(p22;q23)]
	−5, del(5q)
	−7
	abnl(17p)
	Complex [≥3 alterations, except patients with t(9;11), t(15;17), t(8;21), inv(16) or t(16;16)]

Table 4.7 European LeukemiaNet classification. *While all *CEBPA* mutations in cytogenetically normal AML are classified as 'favorable' according to the European LeukemiaNet recommendations, it has now become clear that the favorable prognosis is restricted to those patients with double (biallelic) mutations. AML, acute myeloid leukemia; ELN, European LeukemiaNet. Adapted from © American Society of Hematology, 2010. All rights reserved. Döhner et al [15].

Minimal residual disease

The detection of minimal residual disease (MRD) by sensitive molecular assays for genetic alterations (gene mutations or fusion transcripts) or by flow cytometry has been shown to associate with increased risk of disease relapse [22]. In NPM1-mutated AML, MRD-positive status was recently shown to be a stronger predictor of relapse or death than pretreatment genetic or clinical features [23]. It is currently unclear how MRD measurements are best incorporated into treatment algorithms and whether MRD-guided therapy will improve outcomes.

Prognostic factors in acute lymphoblastic leukemia

Various risk stratification systems have been proposed for adults with ALL. The US National Comprehensive Cancer Network considers the following genetic alterations as markers of high risk: hypodiploidy (<44 chromosomes); t(v;11q23) or MLL rearrangements; t(9;22) or BCR-ABL; or a complex karyotype (≥5 chromosomal abnormalities). The absence of all poor risk factors is considered standard risk. Elevated white blood cell (WBC) count (≥30×10^9/L for B-cell ALL; ≥100×10^9/L for T-cell ALL) may also be associated with poor outcomes. The risk grouping used in clinical trials of the German Multicenter Acute Lymphoblastic Leukemia Study Group (GMALL) is shown in Table 4.8.

Risk group	B-precursor ALL	T-ALL
Standard risk	No pro-B-ALL	Thymic T-ALL
	and WBC <30×10^9/L	
	and no t(4;11)/*MLL-AF4*	
	and no t(9;22)/*BCR-ABL1*	
	And CR after first induction course	
High risk	Pro-B-ALL	Early/Mature T-ALL
	or WBC ≥30×10^9/L	
	or t(4;11)/*MLL-AF4*	
	or CR after second induction course	
BCR-ABL-positive	t(9;22)/*BCR-ABL1*	–

Table 4.8 Risk grouping of adult acute lymphoblastic leukemia according to the German Multicenter Acute Lymphoblastic Leukemia study group. ALL, acute lymphoblastic leukemia.

References

1   Swerdlow SH, Campo E, Harris NL, et al, eds. *WHO Classification of Tumours of Haematopoietic and Lymphoid Tissues*. 4th edn. Lyon, France: IARC; 2008.

2   Arber DA, Orazi A, Hasserjian R, et al. The 2016 revision to the World Health Organization (WHO) classification of myeloid neoplasms and acute leukemia. *Blood*. 2016;127:2391-2405.

3   Miesner M, Haferlach C, Bacher U, et al. Multilineage dysplasia (MLD) in acute myeloid leukemia (AML) correlates with MDS-related cytogenetic abnormalities and a prior history of MDS or MDS/MPN but has no independent prognostic relevance: a comparison of 408 cases classified as "AML not otherwise specified" (AML-NOS) or "AML with myelodysplasia-related changes" (AML-MRC). *Blood*. 2010;116:2742-2751.

4   Lindsley RC, Mar BG, Mazzola E, et al. Acute myeloid leukemia ontogeny is defined by distinct somatic mutations. *Blood*. 2015;125:1367-1376.

5   Kayser S, Döhner K, Krauter J, et al. The impact of therapy-related acute myeloid leukemia (AML) on outcome in 2853 adult patients with newly diagnosed AML. *Blood*. 2011;117: 2137-2145.

6   Mauritzson N, Albin M, Rylander L, et al. Pooled analysis of clinical and cytogenetic features in treatment-related and de novo adult acute myeloid leukemia and myelodysplastic syndromes based on a consecutive series of 761 patients analyzed 1976-1993 and on 5098 unselected cases reported in the literature 1974-2001. *Leukemia*. 2002;16:2366-2378.

7   Walter RB, Othus M, Burnett AK, et al. Significance of FAB subclassification of "acute myeloid leukemia, NOS" in the 2008 WHO classification: analysis of 5848 newly diagnosed patients. *Blood*. 2013;121:2424-2431.

8   Vardiman JW, Thiele J, Arber DA, et al. The 2008 revision of the World Health Organization (WHO) classification of myeloid neoplasms and acute leukemia: rationale and important changes. *Blood*. 2009;114:937-951.

9   Bakst RL, Tallman MS, Douer D, Yahalom J. How I treat extramedullary acute myeloid leukemia. *Blood*. 2011;118:3785-3793.

10 McGregor S, McNeer J, Gurbuxani S. Beyond the 2008 World Health Organization classification: the role of the hematopathology laboratory in the diagnosis and management of acute lymphoblastic leukemia. *Semin Diagn Pathol*. 2012;29:2-11.

11 Roberts KG, Morin RD, Zhang J, et al. Genetic alterations activating kinase and cytokine receptor signaling in high-risk acute lymphoblastic leukemia. *Cancer Cell*. 2012;22:153-166.

12 Bene MC, Castoldi G, Knapp W, et al. Proposals for the immunological classification of acute leukemias. European Group for the Immunological Characterization of Leukemias (EGIL). *Leukemia*. 1995;9:1783-1786.

13 Grimwade D, Hills RK, Moorman AV, et al. Refinement of cytogenetic classification in acute myeloid leukemia: determination of prognostic significance of rare recurring chromosomal abnormalities among 5876 younger adult patients treated in the United Kingdom Medical Research Council trials. *Blood*. 2010;116:354-365.

14 Mrózek K, Marcucci G, Nicolet D, et al. Prognostic significance of the European LeukemiaNet standardized system for reporting cytogenetic and molecular alterations in adults with acute myeloid leukemia. *J Clin Oncol*. 2012;30:4515-4523.

15 Döhner H, Estey EH, Amadori S, et al. Diagnosis and management of acute myeloid leukemia in adults: recommendations from an international expert panel, on behalf of the European LeukemiaNet. *Blood*. 2010;115:453-474.

16 Dufour A, Schneider F, Metzeler K, et al. Acute myeloid leukemia with biallelic CEBPA gene mutations and normal karyotype represents a distinct genetic entity associated with a favorable clinical outcome. *J Clin Oncol*. 2010;28:570-577.

17 Döhner H, Weisdorf DJ, Bloomfield CD. Acute Myeloid Leukemia. *N Engl J Med*. 2015;373: 1136-1152.

18 Roug AS, Hansen MC, Nederby L, Hokland P. Diagnosing and following adult patients with acute myeloid leukaemia in the genomic age. *Br J Haematol*. 2014;167:162-176.

19 Haferlach T. How does one work-up an acute myeloid leukemia patient in the molecular era? http://learningcenter.ehaweb.org/eha/2015/20th/103570/torsten.haferlach.how.does.one. work.up.an.aml.patient.in.the.molecular.era.html?f=m6t1576. Accessed August 12, 2016.

20 Klepin HD. Geriatric perspective: how to assess fitness for chemotherapy in acute myeloid leukemia. *Hematology Am Soc Hematol Educ Program*. 2014;2014:8-13.

21 Krug U, Röllig C, Koschmieder A, et al. Complete remission and early death after intensive chemotherapy in patients aged 60 years or older with acute myeloid leukaemia: a web-based application for prediction of outcomes. *Lancet*. 2010;376:2000-2008.

22 Grimwade D, Freeman SD. Defining minimal residual disease in acute myeloid leukemia: which platforms are ready for "prime time"? *Blood*. 2014;124:3345-3355.

23 Ivey A, Hills RK, Simpson MA, et al. Assessment of minimal residual disease in standard-risk AML. *N Engl J Med*. 2016;374:422-433.

Chapter 5

Therapeutic management of acute myeloid leukemia

Michael Fiegl

Overview of treatment options

Acute myeloid leukemia (AML) is considered a curable disease and hence the primary therapeutic intention in a patient with newly diagnosed AML should be to cure the patient with intensive chemotherapy. However, there are two main reasons why clinicians should not follow this approach: firstly, intensive chemotherapy cannot be administered safely due to comorbidities (or patient refusal), and secondly, the patient will not benefit from intensive chemotherapy because of high-risk AML, which requires allogeneic stem cell transplantation that cannot be performed because of advanced age, comorbidities, or patient refusal. Such patients will receive palliative care as a cure is not achievable. Importantly, advanced age alone is no reason for withholding intensive chemotherapy.

Treatment by phase

Intensive chemotherapy with curative intention is divided into two stages: first, remission induction therapy, which is then followed by post-remission therapy [1]. Post-remission therapy may comprise conventional chemotherapy, namely consolidation therapy and sometimes maintenance therapy, or allogeneic stem cell transplantation. While the choice of induction chemotherapy is largely unaffected by the individual

© Springer International Publishing Switzerland 2016
W. Hiddemann (ed.), *Handbook of Acute Leukemia*,
DOI 10.1007/978-3-319-26772-2_5

risk of the patient, post-remission therapy is determined mainly by the genetic risk and the response to induction therapy. This chapter describes treatment options that are considered 'standard' at the time of writing, while novel options are described in detail in Chapter 8.

Remission induction

For over four decades, the backbone of AML induction chemotherapy has been the antimetabolite cytarabine in combination with an anthracycline. The ancestor of this combination is the so-called '7+3', which is still widely used and can be considered a worldwide standard. An abundance of modifications of this regimen exist, with different dosages of cytarabine, different anthracyclines with different dosages, and also the addition of other antileukemic drugs.

Due to the strict correlation of cytarabine with leukemic cell killing in vitro, one aim was to increase individual exposure of cytarabine. This can be achieved by prolonged or continuous intravenous (IV) applications versus applications twice daily, or by increasing the individual dosage (<100 mg/m² low-dose cytarabine; $100–200$ mg/m²: standard-dose or intermediate-dose cytarabine; and ≥ 500 mg/m² high-dose cytarabine [HiDAC]), however cytarabine doses exceeding 1 g/m² (individual dose) might increase toxicity without additional antileukemic effects [2].

While anthracyclines are a fundamental part of induction chemotherapy, there seems to be no relevant difference in terms of antileukemic activity between different members of this group. Although earlier trials suggested such a difference in favor of idarubicine, the dose of the comparator daunorubicin was 45 mg/m² and thus too low [3,4]. Adequate dosage of daunorubicin is however paramount and even older patients profit from daunorobicin without increase in relevant toxicities [5]. Current evidence suggests however that doses >60 mg daunorubicin do not further improve the overall outcome [6].

The addition of a third antileukemic drug has not convincingly improved the efficacy of induction chemotherapy, may it be a cytotoxic drug (for example, etoposide [7]) or a differentiating agent (for example, all trans retinoic acid [ATRA] [8]). The role of biologicals is unclear to date and the addition of these drugs to induction chemotherapy has yielded unequivocal results for example, the addition of tyrosine kinase inhibitor (TKI) sorafenib to induction chemotherapy did not improve clinical outcome in elderly patients [9], but prolonged relapse free-survival in younger patients without affecting survival [10]. While promising, no general recommendation for the use of any of these drugs during induction chemotherapy can be given. Whether this might differ in certain subgroups or for novel TKIs is subject to investigation.

Usually, two cycles of chemotherapy are applied within 21 days, resulting in the so-called 'double induction'. A bone marrow aspirate is usually performed between the two, and while some experts recommend omitting the second cycle if less than 5–10% blasts are detected in this control (a so-called 'adequate blast clearance'), others do so only in elderly patients (≥60–65 years). A dose-dense approach, where the second cycle of induction chemotherapy is given shortly after the first ('S-HAM') has been shown to be of benefit due to shortened cytopenia

Regimen	Drugs and dosage
7+3 [12]	Cytarabine 100 mg/m^2 CI days 1–7
	Daunorubicin 60 mg/m^2 IV days 3–5
modified 7+3 [5]	Cytarabine 200 mg/m^2 CI days 1–7
	Daunorubicin 90 mg/m^2 IV days 1–3
TAD-9 [13]	Thioguanine 100 mg/m^2 PO days 3–9
	Cytarabine 100 mg/m^2 CI days 1–2
	Cytarabine 2 x 100 mg/m^2 IV days 3–8
	Daunorubicin 60 mg/m^2 IV days 3–5
HAM [13]	Cytarabin 2 x 1000 mg/m^2 IV days 1–3
	Mitoxantron 10 mg/m^2 IV days 3–5
S-HAM* [11]	Cytarabine 2 x 1000 mg/m^2 IV days 1–2 and days 8–9
	Mitoxantrone 10 mg/m^2 IV days 3–4 and days 10–11
ICE [8]	Idarubicin 12 mg/m^2 IV days 1+3
	Cytarabine 100 mg/m^2 CI days 1–5
	Etoposide 100 mg IV days 1+3

Table 5.1 Induction chemotherapy for acute myeloid leukemia. A second cycle (similar or different from the first one) may be applied 3 weeks after initiation of the first cycle with the exception of S-HAM, where both cycles are given within 11 days. *G-CSF recommended in patients with adequate blast clearance in post-reatment aplasia. CI, continuous infusion; G-CSF, granulocyte-colony stimulating factor; ICE, ifosfamide, carboplatin, etopside; IV, intravenous; PO, orally; S-HAM, sequential high-dose cytarabine, mitoxantrone, and pegfilgrastim; TAD-9, 6-thioguanine, cytarabine, and daunorubicin.

[11]. Different examples of regimens for intensive induction chemotherapy are listed in Table 5.1. While most of these regimens have not been tested head-to-head, clinical evidence suggests that none of the applied regimens yields better results than the conventional '7+3' in terms of complete remission (CR) rates and survival parameters [12].

Based on these results, the minimal requirements for induction chemotherapy in AML are the combination of cytarabine with an anthracycline and the application of two cycles of chemotherapy (at least if residual blasts are detected in the control bone marrow aspiration 1 week after the first cycle). At least one cycle should contain HiDAC (possibly not exceeding 1 g/m² per individual dose); if two intermediate doses of cytarabine are given, then HiDAC should be scheduled for consolidation. Anthracyclines need to be administered in an appropriate dose, for example, ≥ 60 mg/m² for daunorubicin (also in older patients).

Supportive therapy

For patients who initially present with (hyper-)leukocytosis, it may be necessary to carry out therapeutic leukapheresis. There is no clear threshold for the leukocyte count, which requires leukapheresis but it should be considered in patients with a peripheral leukocyte count >100 G/L and/or who show signs of organ ischemia (for example, increased lactate or troponine levels in serum, respiratory insufficiency, and renal failure). In patients who have hyperleukocytosis but do not require leukapheresis, a pre-phase with cytarabine 100 mg/m² continuous infusion (CI) or hydroxyurea 1 g/m² orally (PO) twice daily (BID) can be administered prior to induction chemotherapy; leukocytes should drop below 30 G/L to avoid or diminish the risk for tumor lysis syndrome. In case tumor lysis is imminent or present, rasburicase 3–7.5 mg intravenously (IV) is recommended.

During and after the application of induction chemotherapy, the patient faces severe bone marrow aplasia for approximately 6–8 weeks. While anemia and thrombocytopenia are treated with transfusions of erythrocytes and thrombocytes, routine administration of granulocyte-colony stimulating factor (G-CSF) is not recommended, as it has no impact on overall survival despite diminishing severity and duration of infections [14,15]. There is no clear recommendation for prophylactic antibiotics during aplasia, however antimykotic prophylaxis with oral posaconazole has been shown to reduce the incidence of invasive aspergillosis [16] and its use is recommended in this setting.

Routine examination of cerebral spinal fluid and chemotherapeutic prophylaxis for meningeosis leukemica is usually not necessary, but can be reasonable in patients with chloroma or AML with monocytic differentiation or neurological symptoms.

Post-remission therapy

After achievement of CR, post-remission therapy is warranted. The principal choice of conventional chemotherapy versus allogeneic stem cell transplantation is made by the individual risk of the patient. In general, patients with a low risk of relapse (favorable genetic alterations) should receive conventional chemotherapy, while patients with a high risk of relapse require allogeneic stem cell transplantation. For patients with an intermediate risk profile, the role of allogeneic stem cell transplantation is less clear.

Consolidation and maintenance

Usually, one to three cycles of chemotherapy are given as consolidation 4–6 weeks after the patient has achieved CR following induction chemotherapy. If high-dose cytarabine has not been given during induction, usually one to three cycles of HiDAC (with or without an anthracycline) are given as consolidation within a 6–8 week span. Table 5.2 lists some examples.

Regimen	Drugs and dosage
HiDAC [17]	Cytarabine 2x3 g/m^2 over 3 hours days 1, 3, 5
TAD-9 [13]	Thioguanine 100 mg/m^2 PO days 3–9
	Cytarabine 100 mg/m^2 CI days 1–2
	Cytarabine 2x100 mg/m^2 IV days 3–8
	Daunorubicine 60 mg/m^2 IV days 3–5
MAC [18]	Cytarabine 2 x 1 g/m^2 IV days 1–6
	Mitoxantrone 10 mg/m^2 IV days 4–6

Table 5.2 Consolidation chemotherapy for acute myeloid leukemia. Usually, one to three cycles of consolidation are given. In the case of TAD-9, one cycle of consolidation is followed by prolonged maintenance chemotherapy. CI, continuous infusion; HiDAC, high-dose cytarabine; IV, intravenous; MAC, mitoxantrone and cytarabine; TAD-9, 6-thioguanine, cytarabine, and daunorubicin.

While the original publication by the Cancer and Leukemia Group B (CALGB) [19], which defined the benefit of HiDAC during consolidation also included four additional cycles of monthly maintenance therapy, this modality is rarely used in AML today despite evidence for the benefit of such an approach [13]. Similarly, autologous stem cell transplantation, which was popular in the 1990s, has lost its importance in consolidation of AML although it might be beneficial in certain AML subsets [20].

Although chemotherapeutic maintenance is not considered as standard therapy, immune-modulating therapy comprising of interleukin 2 (IL-2) and histamine dihydrochloride (10 cycles for a total of 1.5 years after achievement of CR) has been approved in the European Union and can be considered especially in younger patients [21] with a monocytic differentiated AML [22].

Stem cell transplantation

Patients with an unfavorable risk profile are clear candidates for allogeneic stem cell transplantation in first complete remission (CR1). In the large cohort of patients with a genetic intermediate risk profile the role of allogeneic stem cell transplantation is less clear. While for the whole group no clear evidence exist that these patients benefit from allogeneic stem cell transplantation in CR1, there are certain subgroups that most certainly will. In general, patients with an *FLT3-ITD* mutation (and especially those with a high *FTL3/FLT3-ITD* ratio [23]) should be considered high-risk and be allocated to allogeneic stem cell transplantation whenever feasible. Similarly, patients with chromosomal alterations that are neither favorable nor unfavorable seem to benefit from allogeneic stem cell transplantation while those with normal karyotype may not [24]. Patients that display inadequate blast clearance in the bone marrow during aplasia should also be considered as candidates for allogeneic stem cell transplantation as they have an inferior outcome [25]. Ultimately, the decision to perform allogeneic stem cell transplantation in these patients remains an individual one.

Both HLA-identical related and unrelated stem cell donors can be chosen but due to quicker availability and less costs the primary choice will be a sibling donor. Both peripheral stem cells and bone marrow can be used as source with equal outcome [26]. If no HLA-identical or compatible donor (for example, ≥8 out of 10 matches) is available, alternative stem cell sources can be used such as cord blood or a haploidentical donor. The latter seems to equal HLA-identical allogeneic stem cell transplantation in terms of overall survival despite increased relapse rates (and a lower incidence of graft versus host-disease), but less treatment-related mortality [27]. Nowadays, reduced intensity conditioning (RIC) is the treatment of choice, due to equal effectiveness and less toxicity as compared with myeloablative conditioning (MAC). Possible conditioning regimens with reduced conditioning include fludarabine, Ara-C, and amsacrin (FLAMSA-RIC) [28], fludarabine, BCNU, and melphalane (FBM) [29], and 8 Gy total-body irradiation [30]. The increasing use of these regimens has resulted in an increase of the age threshold to above 60–65 years and in selected patients this can even be above 70 years of age.

Resistant and relapsed leukemia

Resistant disease is generally defined as either persistent disease after intensive chemotherapy or reappearance of AML after achievement of CR within 6 months after initiation of intensive chemotherapy, while reappearance of the disease at a later time point is called relapse. While the duration of CR is generally related to prognosis (the longer, the better), relapse itself is prognostically unfavorable.

The only curative option for relapsed/refractory (r/r) leukemia patients is allogeneic stem cell transplantation. While a second CR (CR2) can be achieved in a certain proportion of patients, remission rates are lower than at primary diagnosis and short lived. In the salvage situation anthracyclines cannot be re-applied in the majority of cases due to exhaustion of the cumulative anthracycline dose [31]. Therefore, alternative approaches are applied such as higher doses of cytarabine with its chemomodulation by fludarabine or cladribine or by a sequential dose-dense design. Table 5.3 lists some examples. The relevance of achieving a CR2 prior to allogeneic stem cell transplantation is not clear; therefore if the procedure can be organized quickly, a bridging concept with cytoreductive therapy (for example, low-dose cytarabine or 5-azacitidine) instead of intensive re-induction is feasible.

If the r/r patient is not a candidate for allogeneic stem cell transplantation then the approach from this point is palliative therapy and resembles the one described in following paragraph.

Treatment of the medically unfit and elderly patient

In medically unfit patients, intensive induction and consolidation chemotherapy is not superior to palliative chemotherapy [36]. Hence, while intensive chemotherapy can be applied in certain cases on an individual basis, palliative chemotherapy is recommended in adjunction to best supportive care (BSC). This comprises mild cytoreduction with low-dose cytarabine or hydroxyurea, antibiotics, and transfusions. While mild chemotherapy can induce CRs in a small proportion of these patients, this is usually not possible in patients with cytogenetically unfavorable AML for whom cytarabine was not superior to BSC [37]. Different treatment options are given in Table 5.4. The main treatment goal is to improve quality of life by reducing cytopenias (and hence infections, transfusions, and hospitalization) and to a lesser degree achievement of CR and prolonging of life for the patient. In the course of such a treatment, resistant disease or relapse will eventually arise. In these cases, one of the mentioned regimens might be given, or treatment can be merely supportive.

Regimen	Drugs and dosage
FLA [32]	Fludarabine 30 mg/m^2 IV days 1–5
	Cytarabine* (1–)2 g/m^2 IV days 1–5
FLAG-Ida [33]	Fludarabine 30 mg/m^2 IV days 1–5, 4 hours prior to
	Cytarabine 1-2 g/m^2 IV days 1–5
	Idarubicine 10 mg/m^2 days 1–3
	G-CSF 300 µg/m^2 days -1–5 (+day 7 until leukocyte recovery)
F-SHAI [34]	Fludarabine 15 mg/m^2 IV days 1–2 and 8–9, 4 hours prior to
	Cytarabine* 2x(1–)3 g/m^2 IV days 1–2 and 8–9
	Idarubicine 10 mg/m^2 IV days 3–4 and 10–11
S-HAM [35]	Cytarabine* 2 x (1–)3 g/m^2 IV days 1–2 and 8–9
	Mitoxantrone 10 mg/m^2 IV days 3–4 and 10–11

Table 5.3 Intensive re-induction chemotherapy for relapsed/refractory acute myeloid leukemia. Intensive re-induction chemotherapy in relapsed/refractory acute myeloid leukemia is usually only warranted in patients that will proceed to allogeneic stem cell transplantation. *Patients ≥60 years received 1 g/m^2. FLA, fludarabine and cytarabine; FLAG-Ida, fludarabine, cytarabine, idarubicin, and granulocyte-colony stimulating factor; F-SHAI, fludarabine, sequential high-dose cytarabine, and idarubicin; IV, intravenous; S-HAM, sequential high-dose cytarabine, mitoxantrone, and pegfilgrastim.

Regimen	CR rates (%)	Median overall survival
Hydroxyurea [37]	1	<6 months
1–2 g PO daily		
Low-dose cytarabine [37]	18	<6 months
2 x 20 mg SC for 10 days		
5-Azacitidine [38]	18	24.5 months*
75 mg/m^2 SC (or IV) for (5–)7 days		Improvement over standard: 1.5-fold
Decitabine [39]	18	7.7 months§
g/m^2 IV for 5 days		Improvement over standard: 1.5-fold

Table 5.4 Palliative chemotherapy in acute myeloid leukemia. Both hypomethylating agents (5-Aza and decitabine) have been shown to be superior to standard treatment comprising cytarabine and hydroxyurea (+BSC), but the latter are still reasonable alternatives in selected cases. Effectiveness of the treatment with these agents should not be evaluated before four to six cycles have been administered. *OS for standard arm: 16 months. Only acute myeloid leukemia with ≤30% bone marrow blasts were included. §OS for standard arm: 5.0 months. IV, intravenous; OS, overall survival; PO, orally; SC, subcutaneous.

References

1 Cheson BD, Bennett JM, Kopecky KJ, et al. Revised recommendations of the International Working Group for Diagnosis, Standardization of Response Criteria, Treatment Outcomes, and Reporting Standards for Therapeutic Trials in Acute Myeloid Leukemia. *J Clin Oncol*. 2003;21:4642-4649.

2 Löwenberg B, Pabst T, Vellenga E, et al. Cytarabine dose for acute myeloid leukemia. *N Engl J Med*. 2011;364:1027-1036.

3 Arlin Z, Case DC Jr, Moore J, et al. Randomized multicenter trial of cytosine arabinoside with mitoxantrone or daunorubicin in previously untreated adult patients with acute nonlymphocytic leukemia (ANLL). *Lederle Cooperative Group. Leukemia*. 1990;4:177-183.

4 Wiernik PH, Banks PL, Case DC Jr, et al. Cytarabine plus idarubicin or daunorubicin as induction and consolidation therapy for previously untreated adult patients with acute myeloid leukemia. *Blood*. 1992;79:313-319.

5 Löwenberg B, Ossenkoppele GJ, van Putten W, et al. High-dose daunorubicin in older patients with acute myeloid leukemia. *N Engl J Med*. 2009;361:1235-1248.

6 Burnett AK, Russell NH, Hills RK, et al. A randomized comparison of daunorubicin 90 mg/m^2 vs 60 mg/m^2 in AML induction: results from the UK NCRI AML17 trial in 1206 patients. *Blood*. 2015;125:3878-3885.

7 Bishop JF, Matthews JP, Young GA, et al. A randomized study of high-dose cytarabine in induction in acute myeloid leukemia. *Blood*. 1996;87:1710-1717.

8 Schlenk RF, Fröhling S, Hartman F, et al. Phase III study of all-trans retinoic acid in previously untreated patients 61 years or older with acute myeloid leukemia. *Leukemia*. 2004;18:1798-1803.

9 Serve H, Krug U, Wagner R, et al. Sorafenib in combination with intensive chemotherapy in elderly patients with acute myeloid leukemia: results from a randomized, placebo-controlled trial. *J Clin Oncol*. 2013;31:3110-3118.

10 Röllig C, Serve H, Hüttmann A, et al. Addition of sorafenib versus placebo to standard therapy in patients aged 60 years or younger with newly diagnosed acute myeloid leukaemia (SORAML): a multicentre, phase 2, randomised controlled trial. *Lancet Oncol*. 2015;16:1691-1699.

11 Braess J, Spiekermann K, Staib P, et al. Dose-dense induction with sequential high-dose cytarabine and mitoxantone (S-HAM) and pegfilgrastim results in a high efficacy and a short duration of critical neutropenia in de novo acute myeloid leukemia: a pilot study of the AMLCG. *Blood*. 2009;113:3903-3910.

12 Büchner T, Schlenk RF, Schaich M, et al. Acute myeloid leukemia (AML): different treatment strategies versus a common standard arm--combined prospective analysis by the German AML Intergroup. *J Clin Oncol*. 2012;30:3604-3610.

13 Büchner T, Berdel WE, Schoch C, et al. Double induction containing either two courses or one course of high-dose cytarabine plus mitoxantrone and postremission therapy by either autologous stem-cell transplantation or by prolonged maintenance for acute myeloid leukemia. *J Clin Oncol*. 2006;24:2480-2489.

14 Lowenberg B, Suciu S, Archimbaud E, et al. Use of recombinant GM-CSF during and after remission induction chemotherapy in patients aged 61 years and older with acute myeloid leukemia: final report of AML-11, a phase III randomized study of the Leukemia Cooperative Group of European Organisation for the Research and Treatment of Cancer and the Dutch Belgian Hemato-Oncology Cooperative Group. *Blood*. 1997;90:2952-2961.

15 Ohno R, Tomonaga M, Ohshima T, et al. A randomized controlled study of granulocyte colony stimulating factor after intensive induction and consolidation therapy in patients with acute lymphoblastic leukemia. Japan Adult Leukemia Study Group. *Int J Hematol*. 1993;58:73-81.

16 Cornely OA, Maertens J, Winston DJ, et al. Posaconazole vs. fluconazole or itraconazole prophylaxis in patients with neutropenia. *N Engl J Med*. 2007;356:348-359.

17 Alter BP. Bone marrow failure syndromes in children. *Pediatr Clin North Am*. 2002;49:973-988.

18 Schaich M, Parmentier S, Kramer M, et al. High-dose cytarabine consolidation with or without additional amsacrine and mitoxantrone in acute myeloid leukemia: results of the prospective randomized AML2003 trial. *J Clin Oncol*. 2013;31:2094-2102.

19 Mayer RJ, Davis RB, Schiffer CA, et al. Intensive postremission chemotherapy in adults with acute myeloid leukemia. Cancer and Leukemia Group B. *N Engl J Med*. 1994;331:896-903.

20 Pfirrmann M, Ehninger G, Thiede C, et al. Prediction of post-remission survival in acute myeloid leukaemia: a post-hoc analysis of the AML96 trial. *Lancet Oncol*. 2012;13:207-214.

21 Brune M, Castaigne S, Catalano J, et al. Improved leukemia-free survival after postconsolidation immunotherapy with histamine dihydrochloride and interleukin-2 in acute myeloid leukemia: results of a randomized phase 3 trial. *Blood*. 2006;108:88-96.

22 Aurelius J, Martner A, Brune M, et al. Remission maintenance in acute myeloid leukemia: impact of functional histamine H2 receptors expressed by leukemic cells. *Haematologica*. 2012;97:1904-1908.

23 Schlenk RF, Kayser S, Bullinger L, et al. Differential impact of allelic ratio and insertion site in FLT3-ITD-positive AML with respect to allogeneic transplantation. *Blood*. 2014;124:3441-3449.

24 Stelljes M, Krug U, Beelen DW, et al. Allogeneic transplantation versus chemotherapy as postremission therapy for acute myeloid leukemia: a prospective matched pairs analysis. *J Clin Oncol*. 2014;32:288-296.

25 Kern W, Haferlach T, Schoch C, et al. Early blast clearance by remission induction therapy is a major independent prognostic factor for both achievement of complete remission and long-term outcome in acute myeloid leukemia: data from the German AML Cooperative Group (AMLCG) 1992 Trial. *Blood*. 2003;101:64-70.

26 Anasetti C, Logan BR, Lee SJ, et al. Peripheral-blood stem cells versus bone marrow from unrelated donors. *N Engl J Med*. 2012;367:1487-1496.

27 Ciurea SO, Zhang MJ, Bacigalupo AA, et al. Haploidentical transplant with posttransplant cyclophosphamide vs matched unrelated donor transplant for acute myeloid leukemia. *Blood*. 2015;126:1033-1040.

28 Schmid C, Schleuning M, Ledderose G, Tischer J, Kolb HJ. Sequential regimen of chemotherapy, reduced-intensity conditioning for allogeneic stem-cell transplantation, and prophylactic donor lymphocyte transfusion in high-risk acute myeloid leukemia and myelodysplastic syndrome. *J Clin Oncol*. 2005;23:5675-5687.

29 Marks R, Potthoff K, Hahn J, et al. Reduced-toxicity conditioning with fludarabine, BCNU, and melphalan in allogeneic hematopoietic cell transplantation: particular activity against advanced hematologic malignancies. *Blood*. 2008;112:415-425.

30 Bornhaüser M, Kienast J, Trenschel R, et al. Reduced-intensity conditioning versus standard conditioning before allogeneic haemopoietic cell transplantation in patients with acute myeloid leukaemia in first complete remission: a prospective, open-label randomised phase 3 trial. *Lancet Oncol.* 2012;13:1035-1044.

31 Estey EH. Treatment of relapsed and refractory acute myelogenous leukemia. *Leukemia.* 2000;14:476-479.

32 Milligan DW, Wheatley K, Littlewood T, et al. Fludarabine and cytosine are less effective than standard ADE chemotherapy in high-risk acute myeloid leukemia, and addition of G-CSF and ATRA are not beneficial: results of the MRC AML-HR randomized trial. *Blood.* 2006;107: 4614-4622.

33 Parker JE, Pagliuca A, Mijovic A, et al. Fludarabine, cytarabine, G-CSF and idarubicin (FLAG-IDA) for the treatment of poor-risk myelodysplastic syndromes and acute myeloid leukaemia. *Br J Haematol.* 1997;99:939-944.

34 Fiegl M, Unterhalt M, Kern W, et al. Chemomodulation of sequential high-dose cytarabine by fludarabine in relapsed or refractory acute myeloid leukemia: a randomized trial of the AMLCG. *Leukemia.* 2014;28:1001-1007.

35 Kern W, Schleyer E, Unterhalt M, Wörmann B, Büchner T, Hiddemann W. High antileukemic activity of sequential high dose cytosine arabinoside and mitoxantrone in patients with refractory acute leukemias. Results of a clinical phase II study. *Cancer.* 1997;79:59-68.

36 Quintas-Cardama A, Ravandi F, Liu-Dumlao T, et al. Epigenetic therapy is associated with similar survival compared with intensive chemotherapy in older patients with newly diagnosed acute myeloid leukemia. *Blood.* 2012;120:4840-4845.

37 Burnett AK, Milligan D, Prentice AG, et al. A comparison of low-dose cytarabine and hydroxyurea with or without all-trans retinoic acid for acute myeloid leukemia and high-risk myelodysplastic syndrome in patients not considered fit for intensive treatment. *Cancer.* 2007;109:1114-1124.

38 Fenaux P, Mufti GJ, Hellström-Lindberg E, et al. Azacitidine prolongs overall survival compared with conventional care regimens in elderly patients with low bone marrow blast count acute myeloid leukemia. *J Clin Oncol.* 2010;28:562-569.

39 Kantarjian HM, Thomas XG, Dmoszynska A, et al. Multicenter, randomized, open-label, phase III trial of decitabine versus patient choice, with physician advice, of either supportive care or low-dose cytarabine for the treatment of older patients with newly diagnosed acute myeloid leukemia. *J Clin Oncol.* 2012;30:2670-2677.

Chapter 6

Therapeutic management of acute promyelocytic leukemia

Karsten Spiekermann

Overview of treatment options

Appropriate treatment of acute promyelocytic leukemia (APL) requires genetic confirmation of the diagnosis by fluorescence in situ hybridization (FISH) or polymerase chain reaction (PCR) (promyelocytic leukemia/retinoic acid receptor [PML-RAR+]) and should be performed in specialized centers with experience in APL treatment. The high cure rate of APL can only be realized when therapy is initiated as soon as possible and therefore diagnosis must also be made as early as possible. As pancytopenia can occur in APL, additional coagulation abnormalities such as hyperfibrinolysis should lead to immediate bone marrow diagnostics. When the marrow is packed, smears have to be carefully examined for the presence of Fagott cells. The less frequent hypogranular variant (M3v) has a characteristic cytomorphology and may not be overlooked (see diagnosis information in Chapters 3 and 4).

Once the diagnosis of APL has been established it is mandatory to distinguish high versus non-high risk group patients according to the classification of Sanz [1], which guides first-line therapy. Therapy recommendations according to the German Acute Myeloid Leukemia (AML)-Intergroup are shown in Figure 6.1.

© Springer International Publishing Switzerland 2016
W. Hiddemann (ed.), *Handbook of Acute Leukemia*,
DOI 10.1007/978-3-319-26772-2_6

Treatment by risk group and phase

The combination of all trans retinoic acid (ATRA) with chemotherapy has been used since the 1990s when the benefit over anthracycline (Ara-C)-based induction therapy was shown [2,3]. ATRA induces differentiation

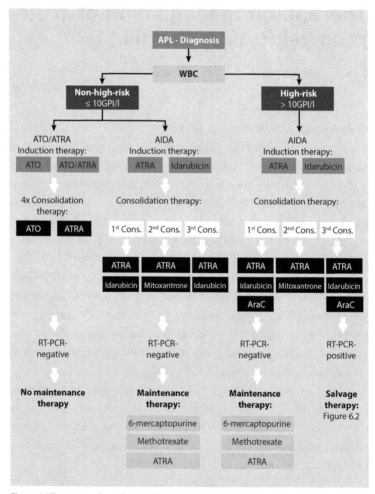

Figure 6.1 Treatment algorithm for first-line therapy of acute promyelocytic leukemia.
Specific anti-leukemic treatment has to be accompanied by immediate supportive management, which differs from non-acute promyelocytic leukemia acute myeloid leukemia therapy (see 'Supportive management' on page 61). Data from [18]. ATO, arsenic trioxide; APL, acute promyelocytic leukemia; ATRA, all trans retinoic acid; Cons, consolidation; RT-PCR, reverse transcription polymerase chain reaction.

of APL blasts, improves coagulopathy, and as a monotherapy can induce remissions in up to 90% of patients.

The European APL group showed that simultaneous ATRA and chemotherapy during induction was superior to sequential ATRA and chemotherapy [4]. One European and US study also demonstrated the benefit of adding maintenance therapy to ATRA [3,4]. Further optimization of induction chemotherapy resulted in the omission of cytarabine during induction therapy by the GIMEMA and PETHEMA groups and established the ATRA plus idarubicin (AIDA) protocol as a widely adapted standard. Further dose reduction in consolidation for low/intermediate risk patients established the current standard of risk-adapted ATRA/chemotherapy, the AIDA2000 protocol (Tables 6.1 and 6.2) [5]. Two randomized trials have established arsenic trioxide (ATO) plus ATRA as an efficient regimen

Group	Year	N	CR (%)	D(E)FS (%)	Strategy
European APL 4	1999	99	94	84	ATRA/DA
GIMEMA [6]	1997	240	95	79	ATRA/idarubicin
North American 3	1997	172	72	75	Maintenance
PETHEMA [7]	1999	123	89	92	No Ara-C
AMLCG [8]	2000	51	92	88	High-dose Ara-C (high risk)

Table 6.1 Early clinical trials comparing ATRA+/– CT and ATRA with modified chemotherapy in the first-line treatment of acute promyelocytic leukemia. Ara-C, cytarabine; ATRA+/–, all trans retinoic acid; CR, complete remission; DA, daunorubicin; D(E)FS, disease- (event-) free survival. Adapted from © American Society of Hematology, 2009. All rights reserved. Tallman, Altman [9].

Group	N	Type of chemotherapy	CR rate (%)
European APL 4	413	Daunorubicin+Ara-C	90–94
French-Belgian-Swiss [10]	340	Daunorubicin+Ara-C	94–99
MRC [11]	120	Daunorubicin+Ara-C+ other	87
GIMEMA AIDA493 [5]	642	Idarubicin (AIDA)	94.3
GIMEMA AIDA 2000 [5]	453	Idarubicin (AIDA)	94.4
PETHEMA LPA96 [12]	175	Idarubicin (AIDA)	90.7
PETHEMA LPA99 [12]	251	Idarubicin (AIDA)	91.1
PETHEMA/HOVON LPA2005 [13]	402	Idarubicin (AIDA)	92.5

Table 6.2 Larger studies using ATRA+CT first-line treatment of acute promyelocytic leukemia. AIDA, ATRA + idaruibin; ATRA, all-trans retinoic acid; CR, complete remission; CT, chemotherapy. Adapted from © American Society of Clinical Oncology, 2011. All rights reserved. Sanz et al [14].

in the first line treatment of APL. The APL0406 [15] and MRC17 [16] trial randomized patients to receive either the ATRA/chemotherapy or a chemotherapy-free regimen consisting of ATO/ATRA. Both trials consistently showed that the ATO/ATRA combination is at least as effective as the ATRA/chemotherapy arm and represents another standard therapy of first line non-high risk APL (Table 6.3).

European LeukemiaNet recommendations

Based on the above mentioned studies therapy recommendations from the European LeukemiaNet [17] were established in 2009 and further developed by national groups for example, the German Intergroup guidelines.

Induction therapy

Induction therapy should consist of the administration of concomitant ATRA and anthracycline-based chemotherapy. Standard induction therapy should not be modified based on the presence of additional leukemia cell characteristics for example, secondary chromosomal abnormalities, Fms-like tyrosine kinase 3 (FLT3) mutations, CD56 expression, and BCR3 PML-RARA isoform. ATO should be used as standard therapy in countries where locally produced arsenic compounds provide a more affordable treatment approach than ATRA plus chemotherapy if these compounds are produced under good quality control. Treatment with ATRA should be continued until terminal differentiation

Study	Patients (n)	Median age (years; range)	Treatment	CR (%)	EFS (%)	OS (%)	CIR (%)	DFS (%)	Median follow-up
APL 0406 [15]	276	45 (18.7–70.2)	ATRA+ATO versus ATRA+CHT	100 97	98 84.9	99.1 94.4	1.1 9.4	98 7.9	36 months (1–75)
AML 17 [16]	235	47 (16–77)	ATRA+ATO versus ATRA+CHT	94 89	91 70	93 89	1 18	NR	30.5 months (3–41.2)

Table 6.3 Randomized clinical trials using ATO/ATRA in the first-line treatment of acute promyelocytic leukemia. AML, acute myeloid leukemia; APL, acute promyelocytic leukemia; ATO, arsenic trioxide; ATRA all-trans retinoic acid; CHT, chemotherapy; CIR, cumulative incidence of relapse; CR, complete remission; DFS, disease-free survival; EFS, event-free survival; NR, not reported; OS, overall survival.

of blasts and achievement of CR, which occurs in virtually all patients after conventional ATRA anthracycline induction schedules. Clinicians should refrain from making therapeutic modifications on the basis of incomplete blast maturation (differentiation) detected up to 50 days or more after the start of treatment by morphology, cytogenetics, or molecular assessment.

Consolidation therapy

Two or three courses of anthracycline-based chemotherapy are considered the standard approach for consolidation therapy, and the addition of ATRA to chemotherapy in consolidation seems to provide a clinical benefit. Consolidation therapy for high-risk patients younger than 60 years of age with white blood cell (WBC) counts higher than 10G/L should include at least one cycle of intermediate- or high-dose cytarabine. The use of ATO in consolidation represents an alternative in patients that have received ATRA/ATO as induction therapy. Molecular remission in the bone marrow should also be assessed at completion of consolidation therapy by RT-PCR assay affording a sensitivity of at least 1 in 10,000. Patients with confirmed molecular persistence should then be considered for allogeneic hematpoietic stem cell transplant (HSCT). However, for patients with molecular persistence who are not candidates for allogeneic HSCT, therapy with ATO or gemtuzumab ozogamicin may be considered.

Management after consolidation

Maintenance therapy should be used for patients who have received a chemotherapy-based induction and consolidation treatment regimen wherein maintenance has shown a clinical benefit, but not for patients after ATRA/ATO based induction/consolidation therapy. Because early treatment intervention in patients with evidence of minimal residual disease (MRD) affords a better outcome than treatment in full-blown relapse, every 3 months MRD monitoring of bone marrow should be offered to all patients for up to 3 years after completion of consolidation. Bone marrow generally allows greater sensitivity for detection of MRD than blood and therefore is the sample type of choice for MRD monitoring. For patients testing PCR-positive at any stage after completion of consolidation treatment, it is recommended that a bone marrow aspiration should be repeated for MRD assessment within 2 weeks and samples should be sent to the local laboratory, as well as to a reference laboratory for independent confirmation. Finally, central nervous system (CNS) prophylaxis should only be considered for patients with hyperleukocytosis.

Treatment of low/intermediate risk patients according to the APL0406 study

Patients are considered to be low/intermediate risk patients if their WBC measures <10G/L at diagnosis. The recommendations as follows are aimed at treating this population in accordance with results from the APL0406 study (Table 6.5) [15].

Treatment of high risk patients (WBC >10G/L at diagnosis) according to AIDA

Patients are considered to be high risk if their WBC measures >10G/L at diagnosis. The recommendations as follows are aimed at treating this population in accordance with AIDA (Table 6.6).

Therapy	Dosage recommendations
Induction	• ATRA 45 mg/m^2 po in two single doses daily until CR, max 60 days • Idarubicin 12 mg/m^2 iv day 2, 4, 6, 8 (only 3 days in elderly and comorbid patients)
Consolidation I	• ATRA 45 mg/m^2 po in two single doses days 1–15 • Idarubicin 5 mg/m^2 iv day 1, 2, 3, 4
Consolidation II	• ATRA 45 mg/m^2 po in two single doses days 1–15 • Mitoxantrone 10 mg/m^2 iv day 1, 2, 3, 4, 5
Consolidation III	• ATRA 45 mg/m^2 po in two single doses days 1–15 • Idarubicin 12 mg/m^2 iv day 1
Maintenance	• 6-mercaptopurine 50 mg/m^2 po daily (day 1–91) followed by 15 days of rest for 7 cycles • Methotrexate 15 mg/m^2 im/po once weekly for 91 days followed by 15 days of rest for 7 cycles • ATRA 45 mg/m^2 po in two single doses daily for 15 days (prior to day 1 or after day 91) every 3 month for a total of 6 cycles; during ATRA therapy treatment break of 6-MP and MTX

Table 6.4 Therapy of non-high-risk APL with ATRA+ chemotherapy according to AIDA.
AIDA, ATRA plus idarubicin; APL, acute promyelocytic leukemia; ATRA, all trans retinoic acid; CR, complete response; MTX, methotrexate; iv, intravenous; po, orally. Data from [18].

Relapse treatment options

Experts from the European LeukemiaNet and the German Intergroup [18] have developed recommendations for salvage therapy of relapsed APL (Figure 6.2), which are available on the European LeukemiaNet

Therapy	Dosage recommendations
Induction	• ATO 0.15 mg/kg iv over 2 h daily starting on day 1; until CR, max 60 days • ATRA 45 mg/m² po in two single doses daily starting on day 1; until CR, max 60 days • Prophylaxis of APL differentiation syndrome with prednisone 0.5 mg/kg day po from day 1 of ATO application to the end of induction therapy and possibly hydroxyurea (see 'Supportive management', p61) when WBC >10 G/L
Consolidation	• ATO/ATRA-based induction therapy is followed by 4 courses of ATO/ATRA-based consolidation • ATO 0.15 mg/kg iv over 2 h daily for 5 days a week; treatment break on day 6 and 7 • 4 weeks on 4 weeks off for a total of 4 courses; last cycles will be administered on week 25–28 • ATRA 45 mg/m² po in two single doses daily 14 days on, 14 days off for a total of 7 courses

Table 6.5 Therapy of non-high-risk APL with ATO/ATRA according to APL0406. APL, acute promyelocytic leukemia; ATO, aarsenic trioxide; CR, complete response; iv, intravenous; po, orally; WBC, white blood cell. Data from [18].

Therapy	Dosage recommendations
Induction	• ATRA 45 mg/m² po in two single doses daily until CR, max 60 days • Idarubicin 12 mg/m² iv day 1, 3, 5, 7 (only 3 days in elderly and comorbid patients)
Consolidation I	• ATRA 45 mg/m² po in two single doses days 1–15 • Id arubicin 5 mg/m² iv day 1, 2, 3, 4 prior to Ara-C administration • Ara-C 1000 mg/m2 iv over 3 hr day 1, 2, 3, 4 after the end of idarubicin
Consolidation II	• ATRA 45 mg/m² po in two single doses days 1–15 • Mitoxantrone 10 mg/m² iv day 1, 2, 3, 4, 5
Consolidation III	• ATRA 45 mg/m² po in two single doses days 1–15 • Idarubicin 12 mg/m² iv day 1 prior to Ara-C administration • Ara-C 150 mg/m²/8h iv day 1, 2, 3, 4, 5
Maintenance	• 6-mercaptopurine 50 mg/m² po daily (day 1–91) followed by 15 days of rest for 7 cycles • MTX 15 mg/m² im/po once weekly for 91 days followed by 15 days of rest for 7 cycles • ATRA 45 mg/m² po in two single doses daily for 15 days (prior to day 1 or after day 91) every 3 month for a total of 6 cycles; during ATRA therapy treatment break of 6-MP and MTX

Table 6.6 Therapy of high-risk APL with ATRA+ chemotherapy according to AIDA. APL, acute promyelocytic leukemia; ATRA, all trans retinoic acid; CR, complete response; MTX, methotrexate; iv, intravenous; po, orally; Data from [18].

website (http://www.leukemia-net.org/content/leukemias/aml/apl).
Patients with molecular resistance or relapse (hematologic or molecular)
should be treated in a clinical trial or according to these guidelines and
documented in disease-specific patient registries.

Depending on previous therapy that the patient has received ATO or
AIDA/chemotherapy-based protocols are recommended. After frontline
therapy with ATRA/chemotherapy, an intensified ATO/ATRA-based salvage
is the treatment of choice. In the case of first-line ATO/ATRA an ATRA/
chemotherapy-based salvage might be used, although this recommendation
is based on expert opinions and so far not supported by randomized studies.

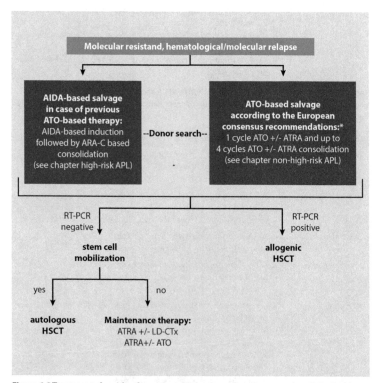

Figure 6.2 Treatment algorithm for patients with relapsed acute promyelocytic leukemia.
AIDA, all trans retinoic acid plus idarubicin; APL, acute promyelocytic leukemia; ARA-C, cytarabine;
ATO, arsenic trioxide; HSCT, hematopoietic stem cell transplantation; RT-PCR, reverse transcription
polymerase chain reaction. Data from [18].

When a bone marrow molecular remission is achieved, patients probably benefit from autologous transplantation. Persistence of PML-RAR MRD indicates a poorer prognosis and an allogeneic stem cell transplantation should be considered.

Supportive management of acute promyelocytic leukemia according to the European LeukemiaNet recommendations

Experts from the European LeukemiaNet and the German Intergroup have developed recommendations for supportive management of APL as follows [17,18].

Leukocytosis

Hydroxyurea (HU) has been used successfully in patients who develop sustained leukocytosis (>10 G/L). It should be dosed to keep the WBC <10G/L and subsequently tapered. For WBC 10–50 G/L 500 mg four times daily and WBC >50 G/L 1000 mg four times daily can be recommended [18].

Recommendations for therapy of leukocytosis according to the European LeukemiaNet [17] indicate that:

- chemotherapy should be started without delay, even if the molecular results are still pending;
- leukapheresis should be avoided due to risk of precipitating fatal hemorrhage; and
- prophylactic steroids can be given, which may reduce the risk of APL differentiation syndrome.

Coagulopathy

The coagulation abnormalities in APL can manifest as a severe hypofibrinogenemia, a prolonged prothrombin time, and thrombocytopenia but also thromboembolic complications.

Recommendations for therapy of coagulopathy according to the European LeukemiaNet [17] indicate that:

- treatment with ATRA should be started immediately once a diagnosis of APL is suspected;
- transfuse liberally with fresh frozen plasma, fibrinogen, and/or cryoprecipitate and platelet transfusions to maintain the fibrinogen

concentration and platelet count above 100–150 mg/dL and 30–50 G/L, respectively; and

- the benefit of heparin, tranexamic acid, or other anticoagulant or antifibrinolytic therapy remains questionable and should not be used routinely outside the context of clinical trials.

Differentiation syndrome

During treatment with ATRA or ATO a differentiation syndrome can develop rapidly and can be lethal if untreated. The presence of one of the following signs should raise suspicion:

- weight gain, peripheral edema;
- dyspnea;
- unexplained fever;
- unexplained hypotension;
- acute renal failure or congestive heart failure;
- interstitial pulmonary infiltrates; and
- pleural or pericardial effusions with or without leukocytosis.

Prophylaxis with prednisone is recommended.

Recommendations for therapy of differentiation syndrome state that [17]:

- steroids (10 mg dexamethasone intravenously bd) should be started immediately at the earliest clinical suspicion of incipient APL differentiation syndrome;
- once the syndrome has resolved, steroids can be discontinued and ATO/ATRA recommenced; and
- temporary discontinuation of differentiation therapy (ATRA or ATO) is indicated only in case of severe APL differentiation syndrome.

Toxicities of arsenic trioxide treatment

Although ATO treatment has a low overall toxicity profile hepatotoxicity and QTc prolongation typically occur, which require dose adjustment or temporary discontinuation. Detailed recommendations were developed by the German Intergroup [18].

References

1   Sanz MA, Lo Coco F, Martin G, et al. Definition of relapse risk and role of nonanthracycline drugs for consolidation in patients with acute promyelocytic leukemia: a joint study of the PETHEMA and GIMEMA cooperative groups. *Blood*. 2000;96:1247-1253.

2   Fenaux P, Le Deley MC, Castaigne S, et al. Effect of all transretinoic acid in newly diagnosed acute promyelocytic leukemia. Results of a multicenter randomized trial. European APL 91 Group. *Blood*. 1993;82:3241-3249.

3   Tallman MS, Andersen JW, Schiffer CA, et al. All-trans-retinoic acid in acute promyelocytic leukemia. *N Engl J Med*. 1997;337:1021-1028.

4   Fenaux P, Chastang C, Chevret S, et al. A randomized comparison of all transretinoic acid (ATRA) followed by chemotherapy and ATRA plus chemotherapy and the role of maintenance therapy in newly diagnosed acute promyelocytic leukemia. The European APL Group. *Blood*. 1999;94:1192-1200.

5   Lo-Coco F, Awisati G, Vignetti M, et al. Front-line treatment of acute promyelocytic leukemia with AIDA induction followed by risk-adapted consolidation for adults younger than 61 years: results of the AIDA-2000 trial of the GIMEMA Group. *Blood*. 2010;116:3171-3179.

6   Mandelli F, Diverio D, Awisanti G, et al. Molecular remission in PML/RAR alpha-positive acute promyelocytic leukemia by combined all-trans retinoic acid and idarubicin (AIDA) therapy. Gruppo Italiano-Malattie Ematologiche Maligne dell'Adulto and Associazione Italiana di Ematologia ed Oncologia Pediatrica Cooperative Groups. *Blood*. 1997;90:1014-1021.

7   Sanz MA, Martín G, Rayón C, et al. A modified AIDA protocol with anthracycline-based consolidation results in high antileukemic efficacy and reduced toxicity in newly diagnosed PML/RARalpha-positive acute promyelocytic leukemia. PETHEMA group. *Blood*. 1999;94:3015-3021.

8   Lengfelder E, Reichert A, Schoch C, et al. Double induction strategy including high dose cytarabine in combination with all-trans retinoic acid: effects in patients with newly diagnosed acute promyelocytic leukemia. German AML Cooperative Group. *Leukemia*. 2000;14:1362-1370.

9   Tallman MS, Altman JK. How I treat acute promyelocytic leukemia. *Blood*. 2009;114:5126-5135.

10 Adès L, Chevret S, Raffoux E, et al. Is cytarabine useful in the treatment of acute promyelocytic leukemia? Results of a randomized trial from the European Acute Promyelocytic Leukemia Group. *J Clin Oncol*. 2006;24:5703-5710.

11 Burnett AK, Grimwade D, Solomon E, Wheatley K, Goldstone AH. Presenting white blood cell count and kinetics of molecular remission predict prognosis in acute promyelocytic leukemia treated with all-trans retinoic acid: result of the Randomized MRC Trial. *Blood*. 1999;93:4131-4143.

12 Sanz MA, Martín G, González M, et al. Risk-adapted treatment of acute promyelocytic leukemia with all-trans-retinoic acid and anthracycline monochemotherapy: a multicenter study by the PETHEMA group. *Blood*. 2004;103:1237-1243.

13 Sanz MA, Montesinos P, Rayón C, et al. Risk-adapted treatment of acute promyelocytic leukemia based on all-trans retinoic acid and anthracycline with addition of cytarabine in consolidation therapy for high-risk patients: further improvements in treatment outcome. *Blood*. 2012;115:5137-5146.

14 Sanz MA, Lo-Coco F. Modern approaches to treating acute promyelocytic leukemia. *J Clin Oncol*. 2011;29:495-503.

15 Lo-Coco F, Avvisati G, Vignetti M, et al. Retinoic acid and arsenic trioxide for acute promyelocytic leukemia. *N Engl J Med*. 2013;369:111-121.

16 Burnett AK, Russell NH, Hills RK, et al. Arsenic trioxide and all-trans retinoic acid treatment for acute promyelocytic leukaemia in all risk groups (AML17): results of a randomised, controlled, phase 3 trial. *Lancet Oncol*. 2015;16:1295-1305

17 Sanz MA, Grimwade D, Tallman MS, et al. Management of acute promyelocytic leukemia: recommendations from an expert panel on behalf of the European LeukemiaNet. *Blood*. 2009;113:1875-1891.

18 Platzbecker U, Lengfelder E, Schlenk RF. Aktuelle Therapieempfehlungen der AML-Intergroup für die Behandlung der akuten Promyelozytenleukämie. http://www.kompetenznetz-leukaemie.de/content/aerzte/aml/therapieempfehlungen/apl. Accessed August 12, 2016.

Chapter 7

Therapeutic management of acute lymphoblastic leukemia

Karsten Spiekermann

General approach for management of acute lymphoblastic leukemia

Treatment of patients with acute lymphoblastic leukemia (ALL) requires a multidisciplinary team and expertise in handling patients, application of therapy, and subsequent complications of therapy such as infections and toxicity. ALL therapy protocols represent the most complex protocols in oncology and treatment in experienced centers is strongly recommended.

There is no accepted standard protocol for the treatment of adult ALL. Therefore, all patients should be treated within a clinical trial. If the patient does not qualify for a clinical trial or refuses enrolment, prospective treatment recommendations from study groups should be followed and the treatment should be documented in disease registries. Detailed diagnosis and treatment recommendations were developed by the European Working Group for Adult ALL (EWALL) [1].

Prognostic factors and risk-adapted therapy

Prognostic factors include parameters of disease biology (for example, genetics and immunologic subtype), patient specific factors (such as age and comorbidity), and response to treatment (for example, time to

© Springer International Publishing Switzerland 2016
W. Hiddemann (ed.), *Handbook of Acute Leukemia*,
DOI 10.1007/978-3-319-26772-2_7

complete remission [CR] and minimal residual disease [MRD] status). The following risk groups can be identified:

- low (or standard) risk group (SR), with a probability of long-term remission >0.50
- intermediate risk group (IR), with a probability <0.50–0.40;
- high risk group (HR), with a probability <0.40–0.25; and
- very high risk group (VHR), with a probability <0.25.

Prognostic factors differ slightly between study groups and therefore different risk models have been developed by the German multicenter ALL (GMALL) group, the Sidney Kimmel Comprehensive Cancer Center (SKCC), the MD Anderson Cancer Center (MDACC), and the Cancer and Leukemia Group B (CALGB). The prognostic factors are summarized in a risk model that estimates the individual risk of relapse and mortality to guide a risk-adapted therapy.

The following risk factors are accepted in most study groups:

- patient: age
- ALL characteristics: white blood cell (WBC) count, genetics, and immunophenotype
- response to induction: time to CR; and
- response to post-induction: early MRD reduction (months 1–6).

Modern treatment protocols stratify patients according to disease-specific risk factors (genetics and subtype), treatment response (CR and MRD), and age. Adolescents and young adults (AYA) represent a group of patients between 15–39 years of age that benefit from pediatric-based treatment protocols. Elderly patients (>55 years of age) are usually treated with lower intensity protocols

Clinical trials supporting current treatment algorithms in first-line therapy

Induction regimens for Ph-negative ALL

National Comprehensive Cancer Network (NCCN) Guideline recommendations for adult patients ≥40 years of age:

- CALGB 881 Larson regimen: daunorubicine, vincristine, prednisone, peg-asparaginase, and cyclophosphamide; for patients aged ≥60 years of age, reduced doses for cyclophosphamide, daunorubicine, and prednisone [2];

- Linker 4-drug regimen: daunorubicine, vincristine, prednisone, and peg-asparaginase [3];
- Hyper-CVAD +/- rituximab: hyper-fractionated cyclophosphamide, vincristine, doxorubicine, and dexamethasone, alternating with high-dose methotrexate and cytarabine; with or without rituximab for CD20-positive disease [4,5]; and
- MRC UKALLXII/ECO2993 regimen: daunorubicine, vincristine, prednisone, and peg-asparaginase (induction Phase I); and cyclophosphamide, cytarabine, and 6-mercaptopurine (induction Phase II) [6].

Recommended pediatric-inspired protocols for AYA patients 15–39 years of age:

- GRAALL-2003 regimen: daunorubicine, vincristine, prednisone, peg-asparaginase, and cyclophosphamide (patients <60 years of age) [7];
- COG AALL-0434 regimen with nelarabine (for T-ALL): daunorubicine, vincristine, prednisone, and peg-asparaginase; nelarabine added to consolidation regimen (NCT00408005; ongoing study);
- CCG-1961 regimen: daunorubicine, vincristine, prednisone, peg-asparaginase (patients ≤21 years of age) [8,9];
- PETHEMA ALL-96 regimen: daunorubicine, vincristine, prednisone, peg-asparaginase and cyclophosphamide (patients aged ≤30 years) [10];
- CALGB 10403 regimen: daunorubicine, vincristine, prednisone, and peg-asparaginase (NCT00558519; in patients <40 years of age);
- DFCI ALL regimen based on DFCI Protocol 00-01: daunorubicine, vincristine, prednisone, high-dose methotrexate, and peg-asparaginase (NCT00165178; in patients <50 years of age); and

- USC ALL regimen based on CCG-1882 regimen: daunorubicine, vincristine, prednisone, and methotrexate with augmented peg-asparaginase (patients aged 18-57 years) [11].

The recommended NCCN-maintenance regimen is:

- Weekly methotrexate + daily 6-mercaptopurine + monthly vincristine/prednisone pulses (for 2–3 years)

Induction regimens for *BCR-ABL*-positive acute lymphoblastic leukemia

For adult patients ≥40 years of age the recommendations are:

- Tyrosine kinase inhibitors (TKIs) + hyper-CVAD: imatinib or dasatinib; and hyper-fractionated cyclophosphamide, vincristine, doxorubicine, and dexamethasone, alternating with high-dose methotrexate, and cytarabine [12,13]
- TKIs + multiagent chemotherapy: imatinib and daunorubicine, prednisone and cyclophosphamide [14,15]
- TKIs (imatinib or dasatinib) + corticosteroids [16,17]

The protocols for AYA patients 15–39 years of age are:

- COG AALL-0031 regimen: vincristine, prednisone (or dexamethasone), and peg-asparaginase, with or without daunorubicine; or prednisone (or dexamethasone) and peg-aspargase with or without daunorubicine; imatinib added during consolidations blocks [18]
- TKIs + hyper-CVAD: imatinib or dasatinib and hyper-fractionated cyclophosphamide, vincristine, doxorubicine, and dexamethasone, alternating with high-dose methotrexate and cytarabine [12,13]
- TKIs + multiagent chemotherapy: imatinib; and daunorubicine, vincristine, prednisone, and cyclophosphamide [14,15]

The recommended maintenance regimen for this population is:

- Addition of TKIs (imatinib or dasatinib) to maintenance regimen
- Monthly vincristine/prednisone pulses (for 2–3 years). May include weekly methotrexate + daily 6-mercaptopurine (6-MP) as tolerated

Results of these trials are shown in Table 7.1 yielding an average cure rate of 35–40% in unselected large adult series from multi-centric trials.

Study (publication year)	No of patients	Median age (years)	SCT strategy	Survival
CALGB 9111 (1998) [19]	198	35 (16–83)	BCR-ABL+	40%, 3 years
LALA 87 (2000) [20]	572	33 (15–60)	All patients*	27%, 10 years
NILG 08/96 (2001) [21]	121	35 (15–74)	Risk-oriented**	48%, 5 years
GMALL 05/93 (2001) [22]	1163	35 (15–65)	Risk-oriented	35%, 5 years
JALSG 93 (2002) [23]	263	31 (15–59)	All patients	30%, 6 years
UCLA (2002) [3]	84	27 (16–59)	Risk-oriented	47%, 5 years
Sweden (2002) [24]	153	42 (16–82)	Risk-oriented	28 %, 5 years
GIMEMA 02/88 (2002) [25]	767	28 (12–60)	–	27%, 9 years
MD Anderson (2004) [4]	288	40 (15–92)	BCR-ABL+	38%, 5 years
EORTC ALL3 (2004) [26]	340	33 (14–79)	All patients	36% 6 years
LALA94 (2004) [27]	922	33 (15–55)	Risk-oriented	36%, 5 years
GOELAL 02 (2004) [28]	198	33 (15–59)	Risk-oriented	41%, 6 years
MRC-ECOG (2005) [29]	1521	15–59	All patients	38%, 5 years
GIMEMA 04/96 [30]	450	16–60	–	33%, 5 years
PETHEMA ALL-93 [31]	222	27 (15–50)	Risk-oriented	34%, 5 years
JOCG 9004 (2007) [32]	143	41 (<64)	All patients	32%, 5 years
GRAALL (2009) only BCR-ABL-negative [7]	225	31 (15–60)	–	60%, 4years
NILG (2009) [33]	280	38 (16–66)	–	34%, 5 years
CALGB 19802 (2013) [34]	161	40 (16–82)	high-risk cytogenetics	39%, 5 years
	8038			27–60%

Table 7.1 Results of modern treatment protocols for adult acute lymphoblastic leukemia. *allogeneic SCT applicable to all patients with potential compatible donor (genetic randomization); **risk stratification criteria vary among studies. SCT, stem cell transplant. Adapted from © Masaryk University Press, 2011. All rights reserved. Gökbuget et al [35].

Overview of treatment options

The following sections will provide an overview of treatment options according to the European Working Group of Adult Acute Lymphoblastic Leukemia recommendations [35].

Chemotherapy and central nervous system therapy

Multi-agent chemotherapy is the backbone of all treatment regimens (with the exception of BCR-ABL+ induction therapy in some trials). In addition, CNS prophylaxis is an essential part of treatment and must be started from the beginning of induction. All patients should receive intrathecal therapy at the diagnostic lumbar puncture. It is a controversial issue whether the diagnostic lumbar puncture should be postponed in patients with high peripheral blast count to prevent spread of leukemic cells to the CNS. Currently available methods for CNS prophylaxis are intrathecal chemotherapy, systemic therapy with drugs that cross the blood-brain barrier, and radiotherapy. The drugs that are in use for intrathecal administration in ALL are methotrexate (15 mg), cytarabine (40 mg), prednisone (40 mg), or dexamethasone (4 mg). These drugs are given either as monotherapy (methotrexate) or as triple combination. In addition, liposomal cytarabine with a prolonged half-life may be used for treatment of CNS relapse. Prophylactic radiotherapy (12–24 Gy) is part of the induction treatment and is administered parallel to chemotherapy in some trials.

Targeted therapies: tyrosine kinase inhibitors and CD20 antibodies

Tyrosine kinase inhibitors in BCR-ABL+ acute lymphoblastic leukemia
BCR-ABL is an initiating event and stable oncogenic driver mutation in ALL. First- (imatinib) and second-generation tyrosine kinase inhibitors (TKIs; nilotinib, dasatinib, bosutinib, and ponatinib) are available and their optimal use in BCR-ABL+ ALL is under intensive investigation. Although no randomized trials have been performed in ALL, retrospective analyses have clearly shown their therapeutic activity [36]. Based on these findings all patients with BCR-ABL+ ALL should be treated with a TKI. In contrast to CML, resistance frequently develops and requires combination therapy and close monitoring. The following general recommendations can be made: (1) the use of second-generation TKI should be restricted to clinical trials or patients in whom mutational analysis suggests their utility; and (2) BCR-ABL monitoring by real-time quantitative polymerase chain reaction (RQ-PCR) is strongly recommended and must be combined with screening for BCR-ABL TK domain mutations in case of suspected resistance.

Recommendations for induction therapy in BCR-ABL+ ALL are that:
- young adults (<55 years of age or those eligible for allogeneic hematopoietic stem cell transplantation [HSCT]) should be treated

with imatinib (recommended dose 600 mg) + chemotherapy (4-5 drugs based induction); and
- elderly patients (>55–60 years of age who are not eligible for HSCT) should be offered imatinib-based induction therapy with the option of adding steroids and/or chemotherapy.
- The use of second-generation TKIs is under investigation in clinical trials.

Recommendations for post-induction and maintenance therapy in BCR-ABL+ ALL suggest that:
- allogeneic SCT is strongly recommended for all eligible patients (sibling or matched unrelated donor [MUD]). Autologous SCT is an option after induction and consolidation in minimal residual disease (MRD)-negative patients and should be followed by maintenance therapy with TKI and/or chemotherapies; and
- for maintenance the combination of TKI and oral chemotherapy is a widely proposed option.

Imatinib does not cross the blood-brain barrier whereas dasatinib does and there is evidence that dasatinib can be effective in treating CNS disease in patients who have relapsed during treatment with imatinib.

Rituximab

CD20 antibodies have significantly improved the prognosis of patients with indolent and aggressive lymphomas and CD20 is expressed in 30–50% of adult B-cell precursor (BCP)-ALL. Very recently, the activity of rituximab has been shown to improve event-free survival (EFS) in the randomized prospective pediatric-inspired Graall-R 2005 Study trial in CD20+ BCR-ABL- adult BCP-ALL [37].

Allogeneic stem cell transplantation

The optimal integration of allogeneic SCT into frontline therapy of adult ALL is currently being actively evaluated in clinical studies. The following risk-adapted indications for allogeneic SCT have been developed by the European Working Group for Adult ALL (EWALL) and are generally accepted for treatment outside clinical trials:
- high-risk conventional risk factors and/or MRD-based risk factors;

- standard risk molecular non-responders;
- relapse including molecular relapse; and
- All patients in second CR (if necessary in good PR or beginning relapse).

Immunotherapy

In addition to conventional monoclonal antibodies such as those that work against CD20 (rituximab) or CD22 (inotuzumab), bispecific T-cell engager (BiTE) antibodies have been developed to engage cytotoxic T-cells for lysis of selected target cells. The CD19 BiTE antibody blinatumomab is composed of CD19- and CD3-binding portions and links T cells to CD19+ ALL cells.

In a pivotal trial, blinatumumab has been shown to eradicate MRD in 80% of ALL patients. This approach has the potential to cure patients, even in the absence of consolidation by stem cell transplantation [38]. Blinatumumab has also shown impressive activity in some patients with relapsed/refractory disease and is currently being intensively investigated [39].

Treatment by phase

The following sections will provide an overview of treatment by phase according to the European Working Group of Adult Acute Lymphoblastic Leukemia recommendations [35].

Remission induction

After diagnosis and parallel to risk stratification the following treatment phases can be distinguished:

- preparative regimen: this is mandatory to prevent metabolic dysfunctions particularly in hyperleukocytotic states, tumor lysis syndrome, and treatment/ prophylaxis of infectious complications;
- pre-induction (optional): corticosteroids +/− other drugs such as cyclophosphamide for disease debulking;
- induction regimen I: patients should receive a four or five drug combination (vincristine-corticosteroids anthracycline-asparaginase +/− cyclophosphamide, or vincristine-

corticosteroids-anthracycline, cyclophosphamide) for 3–4 weeks; response evaluation (peripheral blood [PB]/bone marrow [BM]) should be carried out approximately on day 28;

- early CNS prophylaxis: during induction I with intrathecal drug application;
- induction regimen II (optional): similar to pediatric regimens, this extends the induction period up to week 7 in all patients, and usually consists of cyclophosphamide and fractionated conventional doses of cytarabine and mercaptopurine;
- other: G-CSF to shorten and ameliorate neutropenia from cytotoxic drugs; addition of CD20 antibodies in CD20+ ALL; and
- BCR-ABL+ ALL and Burkitt/B-cell ALL: treatment with highly specific elements is required.

Consolidation

- Chemotherapy: essential backbone that must follow clinical study or current national or international treatment programs;
- CNS prophylaxis: treatment has to include intrathecal therapies and systemic therapies that penetrate the blood-CNS barrier;
- risk-oriented therapy: chemotherapy or allogeneic transplantation based on pre- and postdiagnostic (for example, MRD risk factors); response monitoring must be performed to detect early or impending relapse (MRD); and
- complications: prophylaxis, early diagnosis, and vigorous treatment of infectious complications to reduce therapy-related mortality.

Maintenance

Maintenance therapy represents a standard treatment of adult ALL with the exception of patients with mature B-ALL. A total treatment duration of 2 years with a corresponding length of maintenance is used in the majority of study groups. MRD should be regularly analyzed with validated methods to identify and treat molecular relapse. Maintenance after allogeneic SCT is not recommended (the only exception to this is for *BCR-ABL*-positive ALL).

References

1   European Working Group for Adult ALL. Recommendations of the European Working Group for Adult ALL (2011). http://www.leukemia-net.org/content/leukemias/all/standards_and_sop/index_eng.html. Accessed August 12, 2016.

2   Larson RA, Dodge RK, Burns CP, et al. A five-drug remission induction regimen with intensive consolidation for adults with acute lymphoblastic leukemia: cancer and leukemia group B study 8811. *Blood*. 1995;85:2025-2037.

3   Linker C, Damon L, Ries C, Navarro W. Intensified and shortened cyclical chemotherapy for adult acute lymphoblastic leukemia. *J Clin Oncol*. 2002;20:2464-2471.

4   Kantarjian H, Thomas D, O'Brien S, et al. Long-term follow-up results of hyperfractionated cyclophosphamide, vincristine, doxorubicin, and dexamethasone (Hyper-CVAD), a dose-intensive regimen, in adult acute lymphocytic leukemia. *Cancer*. 2004;101:2788-2801.

5   Thomas DA, O'Brien S, Faderl S, et al. Chemoimmunotherapy with a modified hyper-CVAD and rituximab regimen improves outcome in de novo Philadelphia chromosome-negative precursor B-lineage acute lymphoblastic leukemia. *J Clin Oncol*. 2010;28:3880-3889.

6   Rowe JM, Buck G, Burnett AK, et al. Induction therapy for adults with acute lymphoblastic leukemia: results of more than 1500 patients from the international ALL trial: MRC UKALL XII/ECOG E2993. *Blood*. 2005;106:3760-3767.

7   Huguet F, Leguay T, Raffoux E, et al. Pediatric-inspired therapy in adults with Philadelphia chromosome-negative acute lymphoblastic leukemia: the GRAALL-2003 study. *J Clin Oncol*. 2009;27:911-918.

8   Seibel NL, Steinherz PG, Sather HN, et al. Early postinduction intensification therapy improves survival for children and adolescents with high-risk acute lymphoblastic leukemia: a report from the Children's Oncology Group. *Blood*. 2008;111:2548-2555.

9   Nachman JB, La MK, Hunger SP, et al. Young adults with acute lymphoblastic leukemia have an excellent outcome with chemotherapy alone and benefit from intensive postinduction treatment: a report from the children's oncology group. *J Clin Oncol*. 2009;27:5189-5194.

10 Ribera JM, Oriol A, Sanz MA, et al. Comparison of the results of the treatment of adolescents and young adults with standard-risk acute lymphoblastic leukemia with the Programa Español de Tratamiento en Hematología pediatric-based protocol ALL-96. *J Clin Oncol*. 2008;26:1843-1849.

11 Douer D, Aldoss I, Lunning MA, et al. Pharmacokinetics-based integration of multiple doses of intravenous pegaspargase in a pediatric regimen for adults with newly diagnosed acute lymphoblastic leukemia. *J Clin Oncol*. 2014;32:905-911.

12 Thomas DA, Faderl S, Cortes J, et al. Treatment of Philadelphia chromosome-positive acute lymphocytic leukemia with hyper-CVAD and imatinib mesylate. *Blood*. 2004;103:4396-4407.

13 Ravandi F. First report of phase 2 study of dasatinib with hyper-CVAD for the frontline treatment of patients with Philadelphia chromosome-positive (Ph+) acute lymphoblastic leukemia. *Blood*. 2010;116:2070-2077.

14 Yanada M, Takeuchi J, Sugiura I, et al. High complete remission rate and promising outcome by combination of imatinib and chemotherapy for newly diagnosed BCR-ABL-positive acute lymphoblastic leukemia: a phase II study by the Japan Adult Leukemia Study Group. *J Clin Oncol*. 2006;24:460-466.

15 Mizuta S, Matsuo O, Yagasaki F, et al. Pre-transplant imatinib-based therapy improves the outcome of allogeneic hematopoietic stem cell transplantation for BCR-ABL-positive acute lymphoblastic leukemia. *Leukemia*. 2011;25:41-47.

16 Vignetti M, Fazi P, Cimino G, et al. Imatinib plus steroids induces complete remissions and prolonged survival in elderly Philadelphia chromosome-positive patients with acute lymphoblastic leukemia without additional chemotherapy: results of the Gruppo Italiano Malattie Ematologiche dell'Adulto (GIMEMA) LAL0201-B protocol. *Blood*. 2007;109:3676-3678.

17 Foà R, Vitale A, Vignetti M, et al. Dasatinib as first-line treatment for adult patients with Philadelphia chromosome-positive acute lymphoblastic leukemia. *Blood*. 2011;118:6521-6528.

18 Schultz KR, Bowman WP, Aledo A, et al. Improved early event-free survival with imatinib in Philadelphia chromosome-positive acute lymphoblastic leukemia: a children's oncology group study. *J Clin Oncol.* 2009;27:5175-5181.

19 Larson RA, Dodge RK, Lineker CA, et al. A randomized controlled trial of filgrastim during remission induction and consolidation chemotherapy for adults with acute lymphoblastic leukemia: CALGB study 9111. *Blood.* 1998;92:1556-1564.

20 Thiebaut A, Vernant JP, Degos L, et al. Adult acute lymphocytic leukemia study testing chemotherapy and autologous and allogeneic transplantation. A follow-up report of the French protocol LALA 87. *Hematol Oncol Clin North Am.* 2000;14:1353-1366.

21 Bassan R, Pogliani E, Casula P, et al. Risk-oriented postremission strategies in adult acute lymphoblastic leukemia: prospective confirmation of anthracycline activity in standard-risk class and role of hematopoietic stem cell transplants in high-risk groups. *Hematol J.* 2001;2;117-126.

22 Gökbuget N, Arnold R, Buechner Th, et al. Intensification of induction and consolidation improves only subgroups of adult ALL: Analysis of 1200 patients in GMALL study 05/93 [abstract]. *Blood.* 2001;98:802a.

23 Takeuchi J, Kyo T, Naito K, et al. Induction therapy by frequent administration of doxorubicin with four other drugs, followed by intensive consolidation and maintenance therapy for adult acute lymphoblastic leukemia: the JALSG-ALL93 study. *Leukemia.* 2002;16:1259-1266.

24 Hallböök H, Simonsson B, Ahlgren T, et al. High-dose cytarabine in upfront therapy for adult patients with acute lymphoblastic leukaemia. *Br J Haematol.* 2002;118:748-754.

25 Annino L, Vegna ML, Camera A, et al. Treatment of adult acute lymphoblastic leukemia (ALL): long-term follow-up of the GIMEMA ALL 0288 randomized study. *Blood.* 2002;99:863-871.

26 Labar B, Suciu S, Zittoun R, et al. Allogeneic stem cell transplantation in acute lymphoblastic leukemia and non-Hodgkin's lymphoma for patients <or=50 years old in first complete remission: results of the EORTC ALL-3 trial. *Haematologica.* 2004;89:809-817.

27 Thomas X, Boiron JM, Huguet F, et al. Outcome of treatment in adults with acute lymphoblastic leukemia: analysis of the LALA-94 trial. *J Clin Oncol.* 2004;22:4075-4086.

28 Hunault M, Harousseau JL, Delain M, et al. Better outcome of adult acute lymphoblastic leukemia after early genoidentical allogeneic bone marrow transplantation (BMT) than after late high-dose therapy and autologous BMT: a GOELAMS trial. *Blood.* 2004;104:3028-3037.

29 Goldstone AH, Richards SM, Lazarus HM, et al. In adults with standard-risk acute lymphoblastic leukemia, the greatest benefit is achieved from a matched sibling allogeneic transplantation in first complete remission, and an autologous transplantation is less effective than conventional consolidation/maintenance chemotherapy in all patients: final results of the International ALL Trial (MRC UKALL XII/ECOG E2993). Blood. 2008;111:1827-1833.

30 Mancini M, Scappaticci D, Cimino G, et al. A comprehensive genetic classification of adult acute lymphoblastic leukemia (ALL): analysis of the GIMEMA 0496 protocol. *Blood.* 2005;105:3434-3441.

31 Ribera JM, Oriol A, Bethencourt C, et al. Comparison of intensive chemotherapy, allogeneic or autologous stem cell transplantation as post-remission treatment for adult patients with high-risk acute lymphoblastic leukemia. Results of the PETHEMA ALL-93 trial. *Haematologica.* 2005;90:1346-1356.

32 Tobinai K, Takeyama K, Arima F, et al. Phase II study of chemotherapy and stem cell transplantation for adult acute lymphoblastic leukemia or lymphoblastic lymphoma: Japan Clinical Oncology Group Study 9004. *Cancer Sci.* 2007;98:1350-1357.

33 Bassan R, Spinelli O, Oldani E, et al. Improved risk classification for risk-specific therapy based on the molecular study of minimal residual disease (MRD) in adult acute lymphoblastic leukemia (ALL). *Blood.* 2009;113:4153-4162.

34 Stock W, Johnson JL, Stone RM, et al. Dose intensification of daunorubicin and cytarabine during treatment of adult acute lymphoblastic leukemia: results of Cancer and Leukemia Group B Study 19802. *Cancer.* 2013;119:90-98.

35 Gökbuget N, ed. *Recommendations of the European Working Group for Adult ALL.* 1st edn. Bremen, Germany; London, UK; Boston, USA: UNI-MED Verlag AG;2011.

36 Fielding AK, Rowe JM, Buck G, et al. UKALLXII/ECOG2993: addition of imatinib to a standard treatment regimen enhances long-term outcomes in Philadelphia positive acute lymphoblastic leukemia. *Blood*. 2014;123:843-850.

37 Maury S, Chevret S, Thomas X, et al. Addition of rituximab improves the outcome of adult patients with CD20-positive, Ph-negative, B-cell precursor acute lymphoblastic leukemia (BCP-ALL): results of the randomized Graall-R 2005 Study. *Blood*. 2015;126:abstract 1.

38 Topp MS, Kufer P, Gökbuget N, et al. Targeted therapy with the T-cell-engaging antibody blinatumomab of chemotherapy-refractory minimal residual disease in B-lineage acute lymphoblastic leukemia patients results in high response rate and prolonged leukemia-free survival. *J Clin Oncol*. 2011;29:2493-2498.

39 Topp MS, Gökbuget N, Stein AS, et al. Safety and activity of blinatumomab for adult patients with relapsed or refractory B-precursor acute lymphoblastic leukaemia: a multicentre, single-arm, phase 2 study. *Lancet Oncol*. 2015;16:57-66.

Chapter 8

Future outlook for acute leukemias

Marion Subklewe

Emerging therapies in acute leukemias

In the past 40 years our knowledge about the genetic characteristics of leukemic cells has increased tremendously. This has led to the development of new therapeutic modalities acting on different pathways and utilizing various mechanisms. Examples include the *BCR-ABL* inhibitors, which have substantial activity in Ph+ B-precursor acute lymphoblastic leukemia (ALL) and multi-targeted protein kinase inhibitors such as midostaurin, which have improved survival in patients with mutated fms-like tyrosine kinase 3 (*FLT3*) when applied in combination with conventional chemotherapy. New modalities have also been developed for allogeneic hematopoietic stem cell transplantation (HSCT), which still remains the most successful therapy for prevention of relapse in non-favorable risk patients [1]. Moreover, novel strategies have evolved utilizing the immune system to eliminate leukemic cells. These approaches include antibody-based immunotherapy and adoptively transferred cells (adoptive cellular therapy [ACT]) among others.

Molecular-targeted therapies

Major advances in understanding leukemia biology and its genetic landscape have formed the basis for the development of molecular-targeted therapies, ideally tailored to each patient's disease [2]. A therapeutic breakthrough has been the success of the tyrosine kinase inhibitors

© Springer International Publishing Switzerland 2016
W. Hiddemann (ed.), *Handbook of Acute Leukemia*,
DOI 10.1007/978-3-319-26772-2_8

(TKIs) for the treatment of chronic myeloid leukemia (CML), gastro-intestinal stromal tumors (GIST), and to some extent Ph+ ALL. New investigational drugs against potential driver mutations such as *FLT3* or isocitrate dehydrogenase (*IDH*) have generated promising results in clinical trials in acute myeloid leukemia (AML). However, leukemias often harbor multiple mutations and are potentially composed of sub-clones with various mutations, rendering combinatorial approaches, drug dosing, and administrative schedules an open issue.

Molecular-targeted therapies in acute lymphoblastic leukemia

The advent of TKIs has completely changed the therapeutic landscape of Ph+ ALL (Table 8.1). A TKI combined with chemotherapy is now used as the standard treatment for newly diagnosed Ph+ ALL patients. However, development of resistance to first but also to second-generation TKIs (for example, dasatinib, nilotinib, and bosutinib) due to *T315I* mutations are common causes of disease recurrence. Third generation TKIs such as ponatinib might overcome this problem but there are also other molecular targets for combinatorial or alternative strategies [3]. Preclinical data have demonstrated promising efficacy of pan-phosphoinositide 3 kinase (PI3K) and mechanistic target of rapamycin (mTOR) inhibitors against B- and T-ALL cell lines and phase I studies are under way for relapsed and refractory (r/r) ALL. In T-ALL, NOTCH1, a transmembrane protein that is important during normal thymocyte development, has been found to be mutated and translocated in up to 60% of cases. Multiple small molecules inhibiting the intracellular γ-secretase of NOTCH have been developed but unfortunately the first trials have failed to demonstrate clinical benefit [4].

Molecular-targeted therapies in acute myeloid leukemia

Next-generation sequencing has also facilitated the design of molecular-targeted therapies in AML (Table 8.1). Small molecules targeting mutated or overexpressed proteins involved in a variety of pathways have been developed. These molecules act by inhibiting signaling pathways (eg, kinase inhibitors) or cellular functions (eg, regulators of apoptosis)

[5]. *FLT3* is the most common mutation in AML and occurs in approximately one-third of all de novo AML cases. However, first-generation *FLT3* inhibitors (sorafenib and sunitinib) have failed to show sustainable responses as single agents in phase I/II trials in r/r AML. Current developments focus on more selective inhibitors of *FLT3* but more importantly on combinatorial approaches [6]. The relevance of genomic studies is demonstrated by the successful development of IDH type 2 (IDH2) inhibitors after the revelation of recurrent hot-spot mutations in *IDH1* and *IDH2* in normal karyotype AML. The first clinical data from r/r, *IDH2*-mutated AML patients resulted in an overall response rate of 41%. Other agents against molecular targets have entered clinical trials potentially offering treatment options for patients with molecularly defined AML subtypes (DOT1L inhibitor, bcl-2 inhibitor, bromodomain [BET] inhibitor). Currently, it appears unlikely that small molecules will replace conventional chemotherapy in AML but they will rather be integrated into combinatorial approaches with cytotoxic, hypomethylating, or immunotherapeutic approaches.

Allogeneic hematopoietic stem cell transplantation

Allogeneic HSCT is the most promising approach for preventing recurrence of acute leukemia. However, although transplant-related mortality (TRM) has significantly decreased in the past decades, controversy remains about which patients will benefit from HSCT in first remission; in particular, as risk categories are refined and standard risk factors are annihilated by minimal residual disease (MRD) assessment [7,8]. The patient cohort eligible for allogeneic HSCT is markedly growing as transplant recipient age and stem cell availability is increasing. T-cell-replete haploidentical transplantation has recently emerged as a new alternative transplant modality. Prospectively, advances in immunotherapy will empower us with more specific tools to eradicate leukemia-initiating cells responsible for relapse.

Target	Indication	Inhibitor	Phase	Patient number	Response rate	NCT identifier
ALL: examples of published and registered clinical trials						
BCR-ABL	Ph+, <60	Imatinib	III	268	OS 43% at 5 years	NCT00327678
BCR-ABL	Ph+	Dasatinib	II	53	OS of 69%/ DFS of 51% at 20 months	NCT00391989
BCR-ABL	Ph+	Nilotinib	II	91	OS of 72% at 24 months	NCT00844298
BCR-ABL	Ph+	Ponatinib	II	60	NA	NCT01424982
PI3K, mTOR	r/r	BEZ235	I	23	NA	NCT01756118
NOTCH	T-ALL / T-LBL	LY3039478	I-II	92	NA	NCT02518113
AML: examples of published and registered clinical trials						
FLT3	*FLT3* mutated	Crenolanib	I-II	88	NA	NCT02400281
FLT3	*FLT3* mutated	Quizartinib	III	326	NA	NCT02039726
FLT3	*FLT3* mutated, <60	Midostaurin	III	717	23% increase in OS	NCT00651261
FLT3	*FLT3* mutated, *c-KIT* mutated	Midostaurin	II	18	NA	NCT01830361
c-KIT	*c-KIT* mutated	Dasatinib	III	277	NA	NCT02013648
IDH2	*IDH2* mutated	AG-221	I-II	375	NA	NCT01915498
Bcl-2	*IDH2* mutated, other	Venetoclax	II	NA	NA	NCT01994837
BET proteins	*MLL* rearranged, NPM1c, other, NHL, MM	OTX015	I-II	180	NA	NCT01713582
hDOT1L	*MLL* rearranged	EPZ-5676	I	60	NA	NCT01684150

Table 8.1 Molecular targeted therapy in acute leukemia. ALL, acute lymphoblastic leukemia; AML, acute myeloid leukemia; FLT3, fms-like tyrosine kinase 3; IDH2, isocitrate dehydrogenase; LBL, lymphoblastic lymphoma/leukemia; NA, not applicable. Data from clinicaltrials.gov (last update: 03/2016).

Allogeneic hematopoietic stem cell transplantation in acute lymphoblastic leukemia

Several meta-analyses of randomized trials have concluded that allogeneic HSCT with myeloablative conditioning is beneficial for high-risk adult patients with ALL in first complete remission. In contrast, the benefit of HSCT in standard risk ALL is controversial. More recent results have demonstrated the relevance of MRD status prior to allogeneic HSCT. Thus, MRD negativity is able to confirm standard risk in ALL patients with a low risk of relapse. Accordingly, most ALL study groups do not recommend to proceed to allogeneic HSCT in this setting. For the MRD-negative, high-risk group of ALL patients the recommendations are more controversial. In contrast, HSCT is the treatment of choice in Ph+ ALL patients. The combination of TKI-based induction-consolidation chemotherapy and myeloablative allogeneic HSCT has resulted in very promising 3-year overall survival rates in younger patients [9]. Across all studies and all ALL subtypes, the MRD status prior to allogeneic HSCT is highly predictive of relapse. Since persistence of MRD after HSCT is also significantly associated with poor outcome, these patients should be considered for early interventional trials including antibody- or cell-based immunotherapy.

Allogeneic hematopoietic stem cell transplantation in acute myeloid leukemia

Allogeneic HSCT is the preferred type of post-remission therapy in the adverse genetic risk group of AML. In contrast, the relevance of allogeneic HSCT in intermediate-risk AML is still being debated [10]. Recent data demonstrate the high association of MRD positivity and relapse rate at the time of myeloablative allogeneic HSCT [7]. In the future, a differential genetic risk profile in addition to MRD status will most likely guide the choice of post-remission therapy. In principle, increased options for conditioning regimens and donor source have opened up the possibility of allogeneic HSCT for the vast majority of medically fit patients. Double umbilical cord blood donor transplantation is another option for adult AML patients. Most recently, T-cell repleted haploidentical HSCT has shown comparable results to matched unrelated donor (MUD) HSCT with high rates of engraftment and acceptable rates of severe acute graft versus host disease.

In summary, the current data suggest similar results for stem cell transplantation using alternative donor strategies. Although feasibility of allogeneic HSCT is increasing, questions on donor hierarchy and preferred conditioning regimens remain. Moreover, novel post-transplant strategies are needed to modulate graft-versus leukemia effects and prevent relapse. Agents against molecular and immunotherapeutic targets have evolved and should to be applied in the post-transplant setting [11].

Antibody-based immunotherapy for acute leukemia

Until recently, only anti-CD20-directed antibody therapy has been applied as a beneficial additive to conventional chemotherapy in ALL. Rituximab is a chimeric monoclonal antibody directed against CD20, which has been incorporated into treatment protocols in ALL and B-cell lymphoma. Several study groups, including the German Multicenter Study Group for ALL (GMALL) have reported an improvement in 5-year overall survival rates with the addition of rituximab to standard induction and consolidation chemotherapy in patients <55 years of age [12]. Second generation anti-CD20 antibodies such as ofatumumab and obinutuzumab bind to an alternative epitope of CD20 and have been glycoengineered for an increased induction of cell death through antibody-mediated cytotoxicity. Novel monoclonal antibody formats target CD19 or CD22 in the case of ALL and CD33 or CD123 in the case of AML, and are either available as conventional antibodies or conjugated to cytotoxic agents. Novel T-cell recruiting antibodies adopt a completely different approach by serving as adaptor molecules between T cells and leukemic cells (Figure 8.1).

Antibody drug conjugates in acute lymphoblastic leukemia

Inotuzumab ozogamicin is a humanized monoclonal IgG4 antibody directed against the B-cell surface molecule CD22. It is conjugated to the bacterial-derived toxin calicheamicin, which is also used as a toxic agent in gemtuzumab ozogamicin for AML. Upon binding, CD22 is rapidly internalized thereby delivering the toxin into the cell, which induces

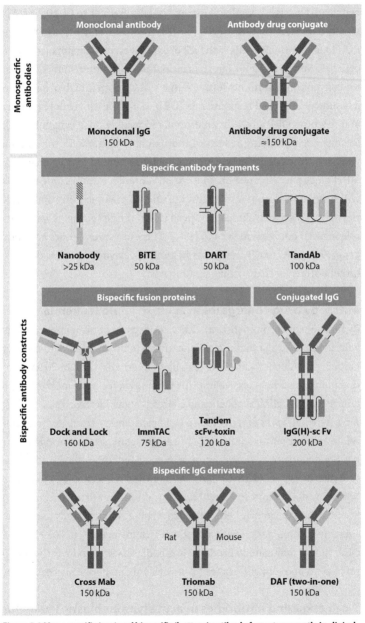

Figure 8.1 Monospecific (top) and bispecific (bottom) antibody formats currently in clinical trials for benign and malignant conditions. Red: primary domain; blue: secondary domain; dark shades: heavy chains; light shades: light chains; green circles: toxin/drug/radioisotope. BiTE, bispecific T-cell engager; DART, dual affinity retargeting molecule. Adapted from [13].

cell death through DNA double-strand breaks. Similar to CD20, CD22 is widely expressed on B-ALL cells (> 90% pre-B-ALL and 100% in mature B-ALL) and normal B cells with lack of expression on hematopoietic stem cells. However, its rapid internalization makes it an unsuitable target for conventional antibody formats. In r/r ALL, inotuzumab ozogamicin has shown an overall response rate (ORR) of 57% as single dose therapy and 59–66% ORR given in an attenuated weekly dose schedule [14]. Despite the promising results of inotuzumab ozogamicin in r/r ALL with two-thirds of patients achieving complete remission (CR) including MRD negativity, the responses were not durable. Future clinical trials will have to explore the role of inotuzumab ozogamicin in combinatorial approaches with chemotherapy in the frontline setting as well as its role in MRD eradication prior to HSCT. There are several other antibody drug conjugate (ADC) constructs in clinical development that differ in target antigen or drug conjugate (Table 8.2).

Antibody drug conjugates in acute myeloid leukemia

By far the most prominent anti-CD33 antibody in clinical application is gemtuzumab ozogamicin, a calicheamicin-toxin conjugated construct inducing DNA double-strand breaks upon internalization. In 2010, gemtuzumab ozogamicin was voluntarily withdrawn from the market due to failure to verify clinical benefit and concerns about increased side effects. Adverse events were attributed to linker instability resulting in toxin-related off-target toxicities [15]. In recent years, a considerable effort has been made to optimize immune-conjugated anti-CD33 antibodies. One such construct (SGN-CD33A) has improved the technology to reduce linker instability and to allow precise and uniform drug loading [16]. SGN-CD33A is currently being tested in a Phase I clinical study as a single agent or in combination with a hypomethylating agent (NCT01902329). Other toxin-conjugated anti-CD33 antibodies have been investigated in preclinical and clinical studies [17], with only moderate success so far.

T-cell engaging antibodies in acute lymphoblastic leukemia

Bispecific T-cell engagers (BiTE) are a novel class of bispecific antibodies in cancer immunotherapy. They are composed of two single-chain

Fv (scFv) fragments, one targeting a tumor-associated antigen, the other binding a T-cell associated surface receptor. Through binding of CD3ε in the T-cell receptor complex, BiTEs are able to recruit T cells irrespective of their antigen specificity. Blinatumomab is the first-in-class BiTE antibody construct targeting CD19 in B-cell malignancies [18]. The target antigen CD19 is expressed in 90% of pre-B-ALL and mature B-ALL patients. In normal hematopoiesis CD19 is expressed at all stages of B-cell differentiation, with the highest expression on mature B cells but little expression on terminal differentiated plasma cells [19].

Target	Name	Phase	Format	Mechanism of action
ALL: published and registered clinical trials				
CD3 x CD19	Blinatumomab	Approved in US and in EU	BiTE	T-cell-mediated cytotoxicity
CD22	Inotuzumab ozogamicin	III	ADC	Toxin-mediated cytotoxicity
CD22	Moxetumomab pasudotox	II	ADC	Toxin-mediated cytotoxicity
CD19	ADCT-402	I	ADC	Toxin-mediated cytotoxicity
CD19	Denintuzumab mafodotin	I	ADC	Toxin-mediated cytotoxicity
CD19 x CD22	DT2219ARL	I	2 scFv + Diphtherie-toxin	Toxin-mediated cytotoxicity
AML: published and registered clinical trials				
CD33	Gemtuzumab ozogamicin	IV	ADC	Toxin-mediated cytotoxicity
CD33	Vadastuximab talirine	I/II	ADC	Toxin-mediated cytotoxicity
CD25	ADCT-301	I	ADC	Toxin-mediated cytotoxicity
CD37	AGS67E	I	ADC	Toxin-mediated cytotoxicity
CD33	IMGN779	I	ADC	Toxin-mediated cytotoxicity
CD3 x CD33	AMG330	I	BiTE	T-cell-mediated cytotoxicity
CD3 x CD123	MGD006	0	DART	T-cell-mediated cytotoxicity

Table 8.2 Antibody-based approaches in acute leukemia. ADC, antibody drug conjugate; ALL, acute lymphoblastic leukemia; AML, acute myeloid leukemia; BiTE, bispecific T-cell engager; DART, dual affinity retargeting molecule. Data from [13,24] and clinicaltrials.gov (last update: 03/2016).

In a Phase II clinical study of ALL patients in hematologic and morphologic CR but with persistent MRD, blinatumomab induced an MRD conversion in 80% of patients after 1 cycle. Twelve of the 20 patients remained in CR after an observation period of 33 months. In December 2014, blinatumomab was approved by the United States Food and Drug Administration (US FDA) for the treatment of r/r ALL after 43% of patients achieved a CR/incomplete blood count recovery (CRi) in a confirmatory clinical Phase II study [20]. Blinatumomab-related toxicities are predominantly related to a cytokine release syndrome (CRS) due to T-cell activation and hypogammaglobulinemia due to B-cell depletion [18].

T-cell engaging antibodies in acute myeloid leukemia

Based on the promising results for blinatumomab in ALL, a similar construct targeting CD33 has been developed for AML (AMG 330). In preclinical studies, AMG 330 recruited and expanded autologous residual T cells within the patient sample and efficiently mediated lysis of primary AML cells [21]. Recently, an international, multi-center first-in-human study was initiated evaluating the safety and dose limiting toxicity (DLT) of AMG 330 in r/r AML. Dual affinity retargeting (DART) molecules are composed of heavy and light chain variable domains of two antigen-binding specificities on two independent polypeptide chains [22]. Recently, a DART molecule targeting CD123, the interleukin receptor alpha, was developed for AML (MGD006) [23]. MGD006 is currently tested in a Phase I clinical study in r/r AML patients (NCT02152956).

T-cell engaging antibody constructs overcome some of the pitfalls of immuno-chemotherapy approaches (for example, toxin-related off-target toxicity) and represent a promising alternative strategy as immunotherapy in acute leukemia.

Chimeric-antigen receptor T cells

Chimeric-antigen receptor T cells for acute lymphoblastic leukemia

Chimeric antigen receptor T cells (CARTs) are genetically engineered T cells composed of an extracellular single chain variable fragment (scFv) fragment targeting a tumor-associated antigen and an intracellular signaling domain (Figure 8.2, Table 8.3). Due to missing efficacy the first generation CAR construct was further equipped with an intracellular co-stimulatory domain (second generation CARs). Third generation CAR T cells comprise a second co-stimulatory domain. A fourth generation of CAR T cells is emerging that is equipped with additional transgenes for cytokine secretion or additional co-stimulatory ligands (Figure 8.2). The most prominent and advanced CAR T-cell constructs target CD19. In multiple Phase I studies investigating CD19 CAR T cells in r/r ALL, CR rates of 70–90% could be achieved. In analogy to the T-cell recruiting antibody constructs, CRS was the most common adverse event related to high tumor burden. In contrast to CD19, the choice of the target antigen in other entities, including AML, will be more difficult due to a more ubiquitous expression pattern in normal hematopoiesis. Alternatively, technological advances are needed, for example to put an inducible suicide gene into the genetically modified CAR T cells [25,26].

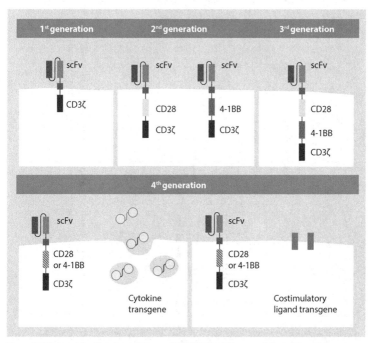

Figure 8.2 Chimeric antigen receptors used for CAR T-cell therapy. Adapted from © American Society of Hematology, 2012. All rights reserved. Brentjens, Curran [27].

Target antigen	Costimulatory domain	Indication	Phase	Patient number	Response rate	NCT identifier	Reference
ALL: published clinical trials							
CD19	4-1BB	B-cell leukemia/lymphoma	I/IIA	30	90% (CR)	NCT01626495, NCT01029366	[28]
CD19	CD28	B-cell leukemia/lymphoma	I	3	66% (CR)	NCT01029366	[29]
		B-cell malignancies	II	10	30%	NCT01087294	[30]
		B-cell leukemia/lymphoma	I	21	60% (CR)	NCT01593696	[31]
		B-cell malignancies	II	15	80%	NCT00924326	[32]
CD19	CD28	r/r B-ALL	I	16	88% (CR)	NCT01044069	[33]
CD19	CD28	r/r B-ALL	I	4	50% (CR)	NCT01860937	[34]
CD19	CD28	B-cell malignancies	I	8	33%	NCT00840853	[35]
AML: published and registered clinical trials							
LeY	CD28	r/r AML	I	4	75%	CTX 08-0002	[36]
CD33	4-1BB	r/r AML	I	1	NA	NCT01864902	[37]
NKG2D		MDS, AML, MM	I	NA	NA	NCT02203825	*
CD123	CD28	r/r AML	I	NA	NA	NCT02159495	*
CD123	4-1BB	r/r AML	0	NA	NA	NCT02623582	*

Table 8.3 Chimeric antigen receptor T-cell-based approaches in acute leukemia. ALL, acute lymphoblastic leukemia; AML, acute myeloid leukemia; CR, complete remission; NA, not applicable; r/r, relapsed and remitting. *Data from clinicaltrials.gov (last update: 03/2016).

Chimeric antigen receptor T cells for acute myeloid leukemia

The choice of suitable target antigens in AML is challenging, as typical leukemia-associated antigens (LAAs) are also expressed in the normal myeloid cell compartment. Kenderian et al showed considerable hematopoietic toxicities in a xenograft mouse model after treatment with CD33 CAR T cells. Efforts to increase the safety profile have been made including the usage of transient expressing vectors [38]. Until today, four Phase I clinical trials have been initiated that study the application of CAR T cells for the treatment of AML including a CD123 CART (NCT02159495). Recently, a safety study evaluating CAR T cells targeting NKG2D ligands has been opened (NCT02203825). Finally, a small study testing a LeY specific CAR T-cell construct has been completed, reporting feasibility and safety of the therapy as well as persistence of CAR T cells for up to 10 months [36].

The success of CAR T cells in B-cell malignancies has shown the potency of this tool for the treatment of acute leukemia. Data in the context of AML are still sparse. Considering the strong on-target off-leukemia effect inherently associated with CAR T cells directed against targets that are not exclusively expressed on AML cells, their application will most probably be restricted to the induction of a remission in relapsed or chemorefractory patients, particularly in the context of HSCT.

Checkpoint inhibitors in acute leukemia

Immune checkpoint molecules expressed on cancer cells dampen adaptive or therapy-induced immune responses through interaction with their ligands on immune effector cells [39]. The use of blocking antibodies against the most prominent inhibitory molecules programmed cell death 1 (PD-1) and cytotoxic T lymphocyte-associated antigen 4 (CTLA-4) has been shown to reverse peripheral tolerance in various clinical trials in advanced solid tumors. These results led to US FDA and European Medicines Agency (EMA) approval of ipilimumab (anti-CLTA-4 antibody) for advanced malignant melanoma [40] and pembrolizumab/nivolumab (anti-PD-1 antibody) for advanced melanoma and lung cancer [41]. However, little is known about the relevance of immune checkpoint molecules in the treatment of acute leukemia [42]. Studies addressing the expression pattern of immune checkpoints in AML revealed low or even no expression of the immune checkpoint molecule PD-L1 [43]. However, PD-L1 was shown to be upregulated upon stimulation with proinflammatory cytokines [43]. The induction of immune checkpoint molecules through targeted immunotherapies needs to be further explored. It is conceivable that novel immunotherapeutic approaches induce immune escape mechanisms that might be suitable for checkpoint inhibitors or combinatorial approaches. Currently, several trials are evaluating the safety and efficacy of checkpoint inhibitors for treatment of AL and myelodysplastic syndromes (NCT02532231, NCT02508870, and NCT01953692).

Conclusions and future outlook

A large number of novel agents are in clinical development for the treatment of acute leukemia. Advances in acute leukemia biology and genetics have opened the door for molecular-targeted agents that act on various pathways and mechanisms. Targeted immunotherapeutic approaches have revolutionized cancer immunotherapy in the past years. Blinatumomab was the first T-cell recruiting antibody approved for the treatment of cancer. Inotuzumab ozogamicin is now being filed for approval. International, multicenter clinical trials using CD19 CAR T cells have been initiated and are currently being evaluated. The success stories of kinase inhibitors, haploidentical HSCT, blinatumomab and inotuzumab ozogamicin, and the promising, albeit preliminary data of CD19 CAR T cells have generated a lot of optimism for the treatment of acute leukemia. Both advanced characterization of leukemic cells and multiple therapeutic tools need to be matched to identify the most suitable therapeutic approach for each individual patient.

References

1   Ishii K, Barrett AJ. Novel immunotherapeutic approaches for the treatment of acute leukemia (myeloid and lymphoblastic). *Ther Adv Hematol*. 2016;7:17-39.
2   Dombret H, Gardin C. An update of current treatments for adult acute myeloid leukemia. *Blood*. 2016;127:53-61.
3   Leoni V, Biondi A. Tyrosine kinase inhibitors in BCR-ABL positive acute lymphoblastic leukemia. Haematologica. *Haematologica*. 2015;100:295-299.
4   Portell CA, Advani AS. Novel targeted therapies in acute lymphoblastic leukemia. *Leuk Lymphoma*. 2014;55:737-748.
5   Reinisch A, Chan SM, Thomas D, Majeti R. Biology and clinical relevance of acute myeloid leukemia stem cells. *Semin Hematol*. 2015;52:150-164.

6   Stein EM, Tallman MS. Emerging therapeutic drugs for AML. *Blood*. 2016;127:71-78.

7   Araki D, Wood BL, Othus M, Radich JP, Halpern AB, Zhou Y, et al. Allogeneic hematopoietic cell transplantation for acute myeloid leukemia: time to move toward a minimal residual disease-based definition of complete remission? *J Clin Oncol*. 2016;1:329-336.

8   Brüggemann M, Raff T, Kneba M. Has MRD monitoring superseded other prognostic factors in adult ALL? *Blood*. 2012;120:4470-4481.

9   Ribera JM. Allogeneic stem cell transplantation for adult acute lymphoblastic leukemia: when and how. *Haematologica*. 2011;96:1083-1086.

10 Gale RP, Wiernik PH, Lazarus HM. Should persons with acute myeloid leukemia have a transplant in first remission? *Leukemia*. 2014;28:1949-1952.

11 Cornelissen JJ, Blaise D. Hematopoietic stem cell transplantation for patients with AML in first complete remission. *Blood*. 2016;127:62-70.

12 Hoelzer D, Gökbuget N. Chemoimmunotherapy in acute lymphoblastic leukemia. *Blood Rev*. 2012;26:25-32.

13 Spiess C, Zhai Q, Carter PJ. Alternative molecular formats and therapeutic applications for bispecific antibodies. *Mol Immunol*. 2015;67:95-106.

14 Yilmaz M, Richard S, Jabbour E. The clinical potential of inotuzumab ozogamicin in relapsed and refractory acute lymphocytic leukemia. *Ther Adv Hematol*. 2015;6:253-261.

15 Lichtenegger FS, Schnorfeil FM, Hiddemann W, Subklewe M. Current strategies in immunotherapy for acute myeloid leukemia. *Immunotherapy*. 2013;5:63-78.

16 Kung Sutherland MS, Walter RB, Jeffrey SC, et al. SGN-CD33A: a novel CD33-targeting antibody-drug conjugate using a pyrrolobenzodiazepine dimer is active in models of drug-resistant AML. *Blood*. 2013;122:1455-1463.

17 Lichtenegger FS, Krupka C, Köhnke T, Subklewe M. Immunotherapy for acute myeloid leukemia. *Semin Hematol*. 2015;52:207-214.

18 Zugmaier G, Klinger M, Schmidt M, Subklewe M. Clinical overview of anti-CD19 BiTE(®) and ex vivo data from anti-CD33 BiTE(®) as examples for retargeting T cells in hematologic malignancies. *Mol Immunol*. 2015;67:58-66.

19 Wang K, Wei G, Liu D. CD19: a biomarker for B cell development, lymphoma diagnosis and therapy. *Exp Hematol Oncol*. 2012;1:36.

20 Topp MS, Gökbuget N, Stein AS, et al. Safety and activity of blinatumomab for adult patients with relapsed or refractory B-precursor acute lymphoblastic leukaemia: a multicentre, single-arm, phase 2 study. *Lancet Oncol*. 2014;16:57-66.

21 Krupka C, Kufer P, Kischel R, et al. CD33 target validation and sustained depletion of AML blasts in long-term cultures by the bispecific T-cell-engaging antibody AMG 330. *Blood*. 2014;123:356-665.

22 Rader C. DARTs take aim at BiTEs. *Blood*. 2011;117:4403-4404.

23 Al-Hussaini M, Rettig MP, Ritchey JK, et al. Targeting CD123 in acute myeloid leukemia using a T-cell-directed dual-affinity retargeting platform. *Blood*. 2016;127:122-131.

24 Chames P, Baty D. Bispecific antibodies for cancer therapy: the light at the end of the tunnel? *MAbs*. 2009;1:539-547.

25 Maude SL, Teachey DT, Porter DL, Grupp SA. CD19-targeted chimeric antigen receptor T-cell therapy for acute lymphoblastic leukemia. *Blood*. 2015;125:4017-4023.

26 McLaughlin L, Cruz CR, Bollard CM. Adoptive T-cell therapies for refractory/relapsed leukemia and lymphoma: current strategies and recent advances. *Ther Adv Hematol*. 2015;6:295-307.

27 Brentjens RJ, Curran KJ. Novel cellular therapies for leukemia: CAR-modified T cells targeted to the CD19 antigen. *Hematology Am Soc Hematol Educ Program*. 2012;2012:143-51.

28 Maude SL, Frey N, Shaw PA, et al. Chimeric antigen receptor T cells for sustained remissions in leukemia. *N Engl J Med*. 2014;371:1507-1517.

29 Kalos M, Levin BL, Porter DL, et al. T cells with chimeric antigen receptors have potent antitumor effects and can establish memory in patients with advanced leukemia. *Sci Transl Med*. 2011;3:95ra73.

30 Kochenderfer JN, Dudley ME, Carpenter RO, et al. Donor-derived CD19-targeted T cells cause regression of malignancy persisting after allogenic hematopoietic stem cell transplantation. *Blood*. 2013;122:4129-4139.

31 Lee DW, Kochenderfer JN, Stetler-Stevenson M, et al. T cells expressing CD19 chimeric antigen receptors for acute lymphoblastic leukemia in children and young adults: a phase 1 dose-escalation trial. *Lancet*. 2015;385:517-528.

32 Kochenferder JN, Dudley ME, Kassim SH, et al. Chemotherapy-refrctory diffuse large B-cell lymphoma and indolent B-cell malignancies can be effectively treated with autologous T cells expressing an anti-CD19 chimeric antigen receptor. *J Clin Onc*. 2014;33:540-549.

33 Davila ML, Riviere I, Wang X, et al. Efficacy and toxicity management of 19-28z CAR T cell therapy in B cell acute lymphoblastic leukemia. *Sci Transl Med*. 2014;6:224ra25.

34 Curran Kj, Riviere I, Kobos R, et al. Chimeric antigen receptor (CAR) T cells targeting the CD19 antigen for the treatment of pediatric relapsed B cell ALL. *Blood*. 2014;124:3716.

35 Cruz CR, Mickelthwaite KP, Savoldo B, et al. Infusion of donor-derived CD19-redirected virus-specific T cells for B-cell malignancies relapsed after allogeneic stem cell transplant: a phase 1 study. *Blood*. 2013;122:2965-2973.

36 Ritchie DS, Neeson PJ, Khot A, et al. Persistence and efficacy of second generation CAR T cell against the LeY antigen in acute myeloid leukemia. *Mol Ther*. 2013;21:2122-2129.

37 Wang Q-S, Wang Y, Lv H-Y, et al. Therapy of CD33-directed chimeric antigen receptor-modified T cells in one patient with relapsed and refractory acute myeloid leukemia. *Mol Ther*. 2015;23:184-191.

38 Kenderian SS, Ruella M, Shestova O, et al. CD33-specific chimeric antigen receptor T cells exhibit potent preclinical activity against human acute myeloid leukemia. *Leukemia*. 2015;29:1637-1647.

39 Chen L, Flies DB. Molecular mechanisms of T cell co-stimulation and co-inhibition. *Nat Rev Immunol*. 2013;13:227-242.

40 Postow MA, Callahan MK, Wolchok JD. Immune checkpoint blockade in cancer therapy. *J Clin Oncol*. 2015;33:1974-1982.

41 Sundar R, Cho BC, Brahmer JR, Soo RA. Nivolumab in NSCLC: latest evidence and clinical potential. Ther Adv Med Oncol. 2015;7:85-96.

42 Armand P. Immune checkpoint blockade in hematologic malignancies. *Blood*. 2015;125: 3393-3400.

43 Krönig H, Kremmler L, Haller B, et al. Interferon-induced programmed death-ligand 1 (PD-L1/B7-H1) expression increases on human acute myeloid leukemia blast cells during treatment. *Eur J Haematol*. 2014;92:195-203.

Printed in the United States
By Bookmasters